PRAISE FOR *THANK YOU, ELISABETH*

"Thank you, Sue, for this compelling and compassionate reminder of the importance of self-awareness and self-reflection to not only serve patients and their families at the end of their life's journey, but also to truly live authentically and be fully present in all aspects of one's life.

Highly recommend this beautiful book."

– MANDY PARRIS-PIPER, PALLIATIVE MEDICINE SPECIALIST

"*Thank you, Elisabeth* is an exquisitely honest and moving account of the journeys a palliative care physician and her patients travel together.

It is an insightful book that highlights the importance of the practice of self-reflection, where there are new learnings in every encounter.

I honour Sue Marsden for the wisdom, insight and experience she brings to the field of Palliative Care."

– LIESE GROOT-ALBERTS, PALLIATIVE CARE EDUCATOR

For Rachael, Michael, and Andrew.

Also, my grandchildren,

and all my other teachers.

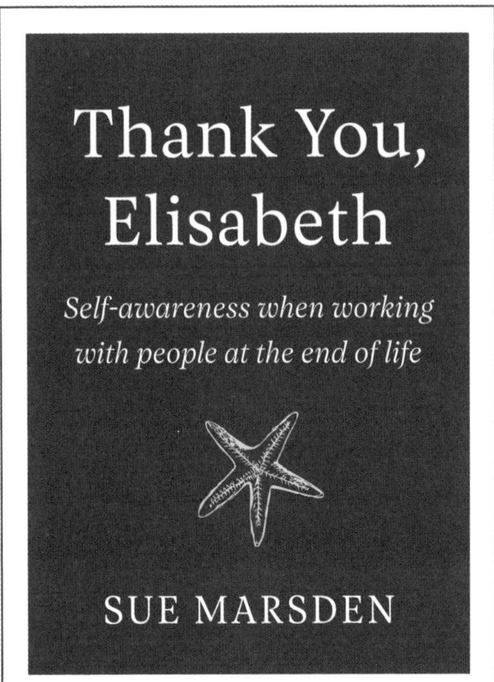
Thank You,
Elisabeth
Self-awareness when working
with people at the end of life
SUE MARSDEN

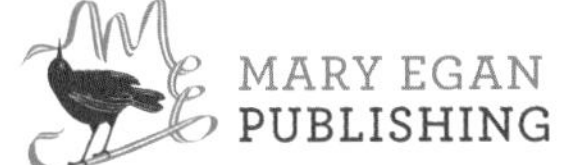
MARY EGAN
PUBLISHING

Published by Mary Egan Publishing
www.maryegan.co.nz

This edition published 2022

Designed by Mary Egan
Cover designed by Anna Egan-Reid
Produced by Mary Egan Publishing
Printed in China

ISBN 978-0-473-62957-1

Contents

Thank You, Elisabeth ...

PREFACE

Palliative care has occupied the largest part of my working life. Inevitably that has been intertwined with my personal life. How could it not be? The longer I have worked with people with life-threatening conditions and those who are dying, the clearer this has become. Who I am, and indeed my whole life from very early on, impacts on how I present myself and work as a palliative care doctor.

These, then, are some stories of my journey working in palliative care. The people I have worked with have taught me much about myself and inevitably changed me forever.

Within these musings are some stories of people I have worked with. Through them I have become convinced that, for those working in such clinical situations, it is important to embrace self-awareness.

It is not my purpose to write a self-help book. Rather, I want to share experiences that highlight self-awareness as a clinical responsibility within healthcare.

S.M.

Chapter 1

MY JOURNEY INTO PALLIATIVE CARE

I found myself back in New Zealand as a senior house officer in 1973. I was in Hamilton and was destined to stay there working at Waikato Hospital for 25 years.

It was my French and German teacher, when I was fourteen years old, who suggested I should become a doctor. I did well at languages but he recognised that they did not impassion me. Medicine did, however, but seemed like a crazy impossible dream. The main message then was that girls get married and have children. But the dream took root and I became determined. After a year at Auckland University studying Medical Intermediate I applied to Otago Medical School. This was the only

Medical School in New Zealand at the time with 120 places available each year. Just a handful were accepted from Auckland. It was such a relief when I managed to scrape in. I headed down to Dunedin in 1965 just before I turned eighteen, naïve and anxious. There were just nineteen women in our class of 120. I recall being told 'You're just keeping a man out of medical school! You'll just get married and leave.' Such was the social opinion of the time. Stupidly, I nearly fulfilled the prediction. At the age of twenty I became married.

I had thought my new husband would come to Dunedin to continue his academic studies. However, he wanted to go to Melbourne. As duty demanded of me, I agreed to go. I had applied for transfer to Monash Medical School but had not heard whether I was accepted.

We arrived in a heat wave and a drought. I thought I was in hell and was miserable because I thought I might have to give up medicine. To my relief, however, I was accepted into fourth year medicine and my dream was preserved. Monash was a relatively new University at the time and had a reputation for rebelliousness. There were often anti-Vietnam war demonstrations outside the hospital. I was quite amused that a good number of the medical students were concerned this might tarnish the respectability of their degree.

After our graduations we spent two years working in Sydney. We had planned to then travel to the northern hemisphere. But my husband accepted a job in Hamilton without consulting me and so back to New Zealand we came.

The only available job for me was a position combining radiotherapy and ear, nose and throat surgery. I was not particularly interested in either specialty. My interest lay in paediatrics.

In the radiotherapy department, however, I met two pioneering radiotherapists, Alan Lomas and Alan Smith. Alan Lomas had been a successful surgeon in Hamilton. He saw the need for cancer services in the Waikato and set about developing the radiotherapy department. He then took his wife and five children to England to train in radiotherapy. Inspired by the two Alans, I was persuaded to train in radiotherapy (now called radiation oncology). I was to be the first to train in this specialty at Waikato Hospital. This in itself was quite daunting.

But then disaster struck. Just four months after arriving back in New Zealand I developed fulminant hepatitis. I had been assisting at an operation and got sprayed in the face by an arterial bleed. The patient was a hepatitis B carrier. I was in a coma for a week. In those days, there was only a 10–20 per cent chance of surviving fulminant hepatitis. But I did.

My marriage did not however.

My two wonderful mentors in radiotherapy were really supportive of my slow intellectual recovery. I recovered physically surprisingly quickly but it took much longer for my concentration and memory to improve.

At that time, radiotherapists also managed chemotherapy. The department would look after patients from the time they were referred until they died. It provided well-integrated and holistic care. My particular areas of oncology interest became breast cancer and paediatrics.

Once I became a consultant, one of the paediatricians and I developed a paediatric oncology service. This was before paediatric oncology was established in New Zealand as its own specialty. There are now two tertiary paediatric oncology services, one in Auckland and one in Christchurch.

Early in my radiotherapy training I met my second husband. A little unexpectedly we started a family and

I sat the exams while six months pregnant. This is not to be recommended. There were, in fact, three lots of exams to get through. As a new parent I quickly had to become much more efficient at studying. I was given some time at work to study but otherwise it was while my little ones were asleep. By the time I finally qualified I had a lively three-year-old daughter and a boisterous 10-month-old son and was learning to be a mother. My second son came about two years later when I was a young consultant. These three young people have been my greatest teachers. They are still teaching me about relationships and about myself.

During the 1980s, palliative medicine was emerging as a specialty in its own right and became such in the United Kingdom in 1987. About that same time, hospital boards in New Zealand were charged with developing plans for care of the dying. A committee was duly formed at Waikato Hospital. There wasn't a huge interest. I volunteered, believing this was important, and prepared a proposal for a palliative care service. The previously dis-interested became interested and opposed the proposal.

A token service was approved in the form of a very part-time appointment. Rather than see this disappear I took on the position alongside my oncology job. I then poured my professional energy into the development of a palliative care service with a dedicated inpatient facility and consultative team. It became a reality in 1990. As a result, the first two trainees in New Zealand in palliative medicine began their training at Waikato.

Just as I was moving into palliative care, Elisabeth Kübler-Ross paid her second visit to New Zealand with her team. I knew I must go the Life, Death and Transition workshop that was to be the focus of the visit. I needed to learn about how to care for the dying from the world-renowned expert.

I was expecting a prescriptive programme and lots of note taking. Was I in for a surprise! We were encouraged to reflect and talk about our own life experiences. This was the beginning of my long and sometimes painful journey of self-awareness.

I quickly became committed to learning as much as I could from Elisabeth's work and so attended many training workshops. Here I learnt about creating a safe space for the externalisation process that Elisabeth taught. This depended heavily on exploring one's own self-awareness. But more about that later. I also learnt to accept honest feedback without hurt and resentment.

And so, consequently, I was honoured to be asked to became part of Elisabeth's facilitating team in New Zealand. For the next four years or so, I facilitated at similar workshops in Australia, the United States and Zimbabwe as well as New Zealand. This not only complemented but also worked well alongside my palliative medicine commitments. When Elisabeth closed down her international organisation, we still continued to do self-awareness workshops for about five years in New Zealand but under a different banner.

The 1990s saw the so-called Health Reforms. As a result, supposed cost-saving measures closed the inpatient palliative care unit. At the time the palliative care unit and adjacent oncology wards were being refurbished. Patients had been relocated temporarily to different parts of the hospital. I was actually on sick leave for some of this time. I was shocked to receive a letter telling me that the palliative care unit would not be moving back.

It would no longer exist as such. I felt betrayed and angry. I discovered too late that the decision had been made based on completely inaccurate information and statistics. Those making the decision had ignored the cost effectiveness of a palliative care inpatient unit.

After living and working for 25 years in Hamilton, I resigned. This was one of the most painful times in my professional life. As my two sons were still at school, for about a year I worked in private palliative medicine practice and at the local emergency centre.

By the end of 1999 I was back in Australia. Here I worked in palliative medicine in a number of settings: inpatient hospice, hospital, as well as urban and rural community settings.

It was in 2000 that palliative medicine became a specialty in its own right in Australasia.

The model for hospice and palliative care services is similar in New Zealand and Australia. The emphasis is on care, as much as possible, in a patient's own home. Where it is not possible at home, the specialist hospice/palliative care inpatient units provide either short-term care to stabilise symptoms or end-of-life care. But inpatient units are not long-term facilities. When a patient is stable and if care at home is not possible, they will be transferred to a rest home facility that provides hospital level care.

While I was working in Sydney, a nurse educator colleague asked for my help with some teaching she had started in the Philippines. The infectious diseases hospital for the poor in Manila had invited her to help introduce palliative care. This began our seven-year commitment, visiting three to four times a year.

About the same time, I was invited to teach at Hospis Malaysia in Kuala Lumpur and became part of their international teaching faculty.

For many years I have had the good fortune to visit Kuala Lumpur annually with my good friend and colleague Liese Groot-Alberts to facilitate a workshop on Suffering and Hope. Liese and I met at that first workshop with Elisabeth in 1987. As well as working together in Asia, we have provided trauma support in Samoa and the Philippines following their dreadful tsunamis.

Whilst working in the Philippines and Malaysia I became part of the Asia Pacific Hospice Network and had the privilege of being the NZ representative on its council for a number of years. This has led to teaching in other countries in Asia, including Indonesia and India.

Moving back to New Zealand once again in 2007, while continuing to visit South East Asia, I provided palliative care teaching and help with programme development in Samoa.

Since 2007, I have worked in several different palliative care settings within New Zealand.

Currently I provide locum cover at hospices as and when required.

What follows are some of the stories of the people I have worked with over the years. Through them I have become convinced that for those working in such clinical situations, self-reflection and self-awareness are vitally important. We owe it to both the people we want to help and our colleagues. We also owe it to ourselves.

Chapter 2

ANNA

Anna looked so lonely. She was lying in a bed in the corner of a four-bedded room. The other three beds were empty.

She was just 35 years old and dying. She had fair skin, blonde hair and a wide smile.

Anna was in the palliative care hospital inpatient unit. She had secondary melanoma, causing nausea and pain that was difficult to manage. She was exhausted. Her husband John and their young children, Marcus and Chloe, would visit, but for just short times each day. This was Anna's wish. She feared the effect on her children of seeing her suffering. She was very clear about limiting their visits.

My role was to manage her symptoms and, with the

rest of the palliative care team, to support her in any way that we could. My routine was to see all patients in the unit each morning.

Like other mornings, this day I stopped at the door of Anna's room. I looked across at her. My gut went into a knot and my shoulders sank. It was a pattern that was repeating. I was spending less and less time with her. Yet what she needed was more time with me.

But my gut seemed to be telling me, 'Stay away!'

What was stopping me from being with this young woman?

At first, I made excuses about having so many other things to do. But there had to be more to it than simply that. After all, my reaction was visceral and quite intense.

I recalled the words of Elisabeth Kübler-Ross at the first of her workshops I had attended:

'If you want to work with the dying, deal with your own shit first!'

Was this relevant to my reaction on seeing Anna?

As I thought about this, it was as if a light bulb had illuminated.

Anna was alone in the hospital room. She looked lonely. I was lonely. I was in the middle of an acrimonious divorce, for me, a very lonely experience. But my loneliness had much earlier roots. As a five-year-old, I had left England with my family and come to New Zealand. I had left my friends and toys and come to a strange new home. My three brothers were all a lot older than me and there were no children my own age living in our new street. I hated it and yearned for someone to play with.

Realising this, released the knot in my gut.

The next time I visited Anna it felt much easier; I went in and sat on her bed. She looked up at me, smiled, gave me a hug and said, 'You look better today!'

From then on, I was better able to support Anna with her feelings and worries, without my own getting in the way.

So often, subconscious issues that have remained unresolved can unexpectedly surface. Elisabeth Kübler-Ross called such issues "unfinished business". When triggered, they can interfere with the provision of support and healing for those we seek to serve.

So, this is what I want to write about.

Self-awareness, I now believe, is a clinical responsibility. I was introduced to this concept at that first workshop in 1987.

Elisabeth had recognised the urgent need for people to start talking about death. This was in the 1960s when talking about the subject was taboo. She also recognised the suffering that occurred when the dying were neither spoken to truthfully nor listened to. She became aware that suffering was increased when the dying were not given the space and opportunity to deal with what she called "unfinished business". So often they were not able to express freely the emotions that had sometimes been pent up for years.

This brave woman set up workshops where, in a safe environment, these emotions could be expressed without judgement and with acceptance. She created a sacred space where emotional and spiritual healing could occur.

Elisabeth then quickly recognised that it was not just the dying who needed this, but that those same things prevented us all from living with joy and peace. Hence the workshops were opened to anyone with grief and unresolved issues. In other words, all of us. One of the powerful aspects of these workshops was having the ill, the dying and the bereaved there, together with health-care professionals.

In my first workshop I heard the sadness and

bewilderment of a woman whose two children had both died of an inherited disease and the anger and pain of a woman whose fifteen-year-old daughter had gone missing five years earlier. I had not, until then, understood the depth of misery caused by loss. Hearing the stories of those telling of bad experiences at the hands of healthcare professionals was humbling. It was extraordinary to observe their relief when, perhaps for the first time, their experiences were heard out loud and thus validated.

For me, having worked for 10 years as an oncologist and now moving into palliative medicine, this workshop was a significant turning point both professionally and personally. I had initially gone to the workshop to take lots of notes in order to learn "how to do it" from the experts in death and dying. Instead, I learnt so much about the power of listening and being present. And of equal importance, by participating, I began my own journey of self-awareness.

I came to better understand the clinical depression I had been carrying since childhood. I met the young frightened girl inside who had learnt to mask her fear and work, work, work to prove some sort of worthiness.

I grew up in an angry household. My father had

multiple sclerosis, and I knew him only as an invalid who was angry and verbally abusive. At the workshop, I was encouraged by the safety that was created. I was able to express out loud the anger of the little girl who was able to tell her father (symbolically — he had been dead for many years) that his illness was not her fault.

The feeling that somehow his illness was her fault came from the little girl's subconscious belief that this must be so. Otherwise, why would he be so angry with her? Consequently, this had translated into a feeling that, whenever anything went wrong it must be her fault. I had never before been able to explain why I always felt guilty. I used to joke that if someone slipped on a banana skin across the road it must be my fault and I needed to apologise.

And so, thank you, Elisabeth, for my first introduction to self-awareness and for showing me the importance of being able to acknowledge that my feelings are real and deserve to be explored, and not be suppressed for being "wrong and shameful".

So often, parallel processes are occurring for our patients and ourselves, as with my experience with Anna. To prevent my unresolved issues being projected into such a situation, I needed to become more aware of these and my own patterns of behaviour. Such awareness could also help protect me from "burnout" and "compassion fatigue".

Most importantly, however, self-awareness would better allow me to be more present for those I wanted to serve.

Therefore, I want to write some of the stories of wonderful people I have had the honour of being present with during the last days/hours of their lives. So many of these people have given me insights into my own issues and patterns of behaviour, and have encouraged my personal exploration of the mysteries of death and, therefore, life.

I wanted to learn how to become more present and authentically responsive to people at the end of life. It seems then that a sacred space can be created for the dying and their families. In such a sacred space, I believe that there is an opportunity for hope and meaning to be experienced, even at the very end of life. My goal has been to better facilitate this.

Chapter 3

LISTENING AND BEING HEARD . . . BEING PRESENT

Medical students usually spend some time in hospices or palliative care units during their training. I often ask them to ask the person they are about to see, 'What is the one thing you would like me to remember when I become a doctor?' Invariably the reply is some variation of 'I want you to make sure you listen.'

By "listen" I believe they mean "pay attention and don't be distracted". I have come to understand that this means paying attention to all parts of the person with my whole being; to be totally present.

Body memory

Cathy

Cathy was 75 years old and nearly blind. She was not imminently dying but had been admitted to the palliative care inpatient unit with uncontrolled back pain, nausea and vomiting. Her back pain remained stubborn to our efforts to control it.

One morning I went into her room and Cathy was curled up in a ball lying on her bed. She looked just like a frightened little girl.

Quietly, I sat down beside her, took her hand and spoke to the little girl before me. I asked her what had happened. Gradually she seemed to notice I was there and tears fell down her cheeks. And the little girl told me her story.

When Cathy was about three years old her mother had died and left her to be cared for by her brute of a father. He was an alcoholic, and was abusive and violent. He would not allow his young daughter to wear underwear, and regularly violated her physically and sexually. Worse, he allowed his drunken mates to do the same. She remembered being violated with beer bottles.

'I've never told anyone before,' she said shyly. She talked on for almost half an hour. Eventually I asked her what her back pain was like right then. She looked surprised.

'It's not so bad right now!' she exclaimed.

We talked more about what it felt like when she had a sudden bout of her back pain and perhaps what it reminded her of. She looked towards me sadly.

'It feels like what they did to me!' She looked surprised.

It was stirring the body memory of her childhood trauma. The concept of "body memory" in the past was not really given credence by conventional medicine. However, there is mounting neuroscientific evidence of its validity. In my mind it made sense of Cathy's pain. More importantly, it made real sense to her. Her pain did not miraculously disappear, of course, but it did become more manageable for Cathy.

My experience with Cathy reinforced how important it is to observe carefully and hear clearly the person I am trying to help. From a medical point of view, she had very advanced lung disease and severe arthritis in her back. We thought she may also have cancer in her gut but Cathy had steadfastly refused to have this investigated. X-rays and scans of her back had been puzzling. Unhelpful. Her physical pain was much worse and out of proportion to what these showed.

To help Cathy, I needed to respectfully and gently connect with the world she was in at that moment. It was as if a sacred space had been created where the little girl within her felt safe. My role was to be totally engaged with that little girl and be completely present.

Hanging on. What keeps us here?

Shirley

When I first met Shirley, she had been in the hospice inpatient unit for two weeks.

We immediately hit it off. We had a similar sense of humour. We laughed together. We swore together. We agreed that what was happening to her was bloody awful and a real bugger.

'I don't think I'll need my vibrator anymore!' she joked. This became quite a focus of our banter.

Shirley had had a hard and traumatic life. She showed

me two tattoos. There was one for each of her dead children. Her daughter had died in a car crash and her son from a drug overdose. How does a mother live with that reality? And, currently she had a daughter in hospital with drug related problems. She described her partner Russell and her eldest daughter, Jane, as her "rocks". 'They have kept me going,' she said.

Shirley had lung cancer which had spread to other parts of her body, including her ribs and liver. She had been admitted with pain but this was now well controlled. She had been described by staff as "super anxious". However, as the days went by, Shirley's anxiety became less of an issue and her physical symptoms remained well controlled. Her sense of humour and playfulness were never far away but she was becoming weaker and frailer. It seemed that she had just days to live.

Because her time was clearly very short it was decided that she would stay at the hospice rather than be transferred to a rest home facility.

Then one day Shirley asked, 'Am I about to die, do you think? I think I will die tonight.'

We talked about her death being close, but exactly when it would happen was hard to predict.

The next morning she described a dream she had had that night. She said that she dreamed she was heading towards a door and that her dead children were beckoning her through. Then a hand touched her arm as if to say: 'No, not yet.'

She was close to dying for several days. What was holding her?

It was a busy day in the hospice unit when her partner Russell suddenly announced that he wanted to take her home and that she would get better.

Shirley had told me that Russell had had problems with severe depression with suicidal tendencies when his marriage had broken up. He had met Shirley and she had essentially rescued him and, with her support, he had been doing well.

I sat down and talked with Russell about his belief that Shirley would get better and not die.

As we talked about his relationship with Shirley and how she had helped him, Russell told me that he had stopped taking his medications about two weeks before. His emotional state was now clearly quite unstable in terms of his mood, behaviour and rational thought.

I pointed out to him that Shirley needed him to be

well and strong right now and that meant he needed to restart his medications. Shirley reinforced this with Russell.

'I'm not going to get better, love,' said this courageous woman, 'no matter how much I want to, or how much you want me to.' Russell looked so dejected but Shirley went on.

'I haven't got long, and you know, I can handle that.' She looked at him pleadingly.

'Please keep taking your pills and get well again. That's what I can't handle — you being in a pickle!'

Together Shirley and I told Russell that the hospice bereavement team would be there to support him when she died.

Shirley died about four days later. She had needed to know that someone would be watching out for and supporting Russell.

There was so much to take on board from the experience of working with Shirley and Russell.

Shirley delighted in humour, even in such dire circumstances, and it was important to share this with her. Also, I was reminded again of the need to hear, without judgement, the stories, concerns and suffering of those we seek to serve. I needed to be completely attentive and present, to facilitate a sacred space that allowed the unfolding of these confidences. And then perhaps it is easier for the dying person to heal and choose their own time to leave …

Hearing the anguish and staying present

Pauline

'Please come and see this woman now!'

My colleague's voice down the phone was desperate.

'You know her and she wants to see you!'

I had known Pauline some years before when her daughter was in day care with my daughter. At that time, she was a solo parent. We hadn't had any contact after the girls had left the day care. But now, six years later she was asking me to see her.

Pauline had gone to live in a country town and had married. She had three more children, the youngest but a few months old. Before she had become pregnant with this baby a malignant melanoma had been removed from her back. It was quite a thick melanoma which meant that it could likely spread at some point.

However, Pauline and her husband told the oncologist that they had understood from the surgeon that it had been totally removed. They had taken this to mean, 'Nothing to worry about.' Hence, they went ahead with the pregnancy.

But . . . disaster. During that pregnancy the cancer had spread and was now involving her liver and bones and causing her considerable physical pain and, of course, indescribable anguish about her children.

I walked into the room.

You could feel the atmosphere. Anger. Fury. Fear. Grief. All came tumbling towards me. Pauline's husband, Martin, was pacing up and down by the window. His face was contorted and his rage palpable. My registrar, a tall strapping young man excused himself, saying he had been called away.

Pauline was lying on the bed grimacing, sobbing and rolling from side to side.

How to help?

Working from basic principles (always a good place to start) I knew I had to manage Pauline's physical pain first.

'We need to get your pain controlled, Pauline. We need to do that first. Then we'll talk.'

And so, with the right medications, once Pauline was more physically comfortable, I sat down on the bed beside her. She was distraught and crying. There was clearly no point in attempting rational discussion about the rights and wrongs of the advice they had received from the surgeon nor what might be possible from now on.

I said to her, 'This is just not fair.' Martin continued to pace and rage and Pauline sat and sobbed. I handed Pauline tissues and sat quietly.

We sat together like that for some twenty minutes.

Martin gradually stopped his pacing and looked at Pauline. He sat down and held her hand. Suddenly Pauline looked up. She grabbed a handful of tissues. She blew her nose and stopped crying.

'Well,' she said, 'we had better decide what we can do about this.'

Now that she was ready, we were able to talk calmly about what could be done and what the future might hold for her and her family.

Another important learning experience. When I

walked into the room, Pauline's pain and emotions were to the fore. I needed to acknowledge that. First and foremost was the need to deal with Pauline's physical needs, her pain. It's very hard to think or deal with anything else when you are so uncomfortable. Next, Pauline and Martin's overwhelming emotional suffering and anguish needed expressing and to be heard.

Only then, when they were ready, could calm and rational discussion take place. Obvious? But how often in healthcare are patients berated when they haven't understood or remembered information given to them because they have, at the time, been overwhelmed with their emotional and spiritual suffering?

What is a miracle?

Miriam

'I will get better. I know it. God will make it happen.' These were almost the first words that she said to me as I entered her room.

Miriam was a 42-year-old woman with a strong faith in her God. She was married with a seven-year-old son, Peter. Sadly, she was dying of very advanced ovarian cancer and her symptoms were such that she needed admission to the inpatient unit for them to be managed.

Her husband, David, was very attentive and at her side as much as possible. Miriam had received exhaustive and exhausting chemotherapy for her cancer. There were no more realistic cancer treatment options available. She would not recover and was dying. However, Miriam insisted that a miracle was possible and all she needed to do was to have more faith in her God.

Peter was soon to turn eight years old and his parents had been planning a birthday party for some time. Was Miriam going to even be able to be there? Today was Tuesday and the birthday party would be the following Saturday. The invitations had gone out more than two weeks ago.

Because Miriam was so unwell and becoming worse quite rapidly, there seemed a good chance that she would not even make the party. Each day, however, she talked excitedly about the party and her beautiful son. It was so important to her to be there.

However, her main focus was that she would be cured of the cancer that was killing her.

David's reality was different.

'What can I do?' he said to me. 'I know Miriam is dying. She needs to accept it!'

'I want to talk to her about Peter,' he continued. 'She won't be around and I want to know more about her dreams for him.'

David was very distressed. He shared her religious beliefs but not her certainty of the miracle cure she insisted on. In fact, he desperately asked us how to overcome her apparent denial of the inevitable outcome. We had no answers.

Miriam's belief was a miracle cure.

All that we, as a team, could do was be available to listen and support both Miriam and David. We encouraged David not to try and force the issue. We tried to give him all the support he needed to be able to just listen and be present for Miriam. This was so hard, when he desperately wanted to ask questions of his wife that she certainly was not willing to entertain. Such discussion would make her upset and angry, believing that his faith was not strong enough.

At times, with David present, I would, as gently as I could, ask Miriam what it would be like if the miracle she was seeking did not happen in the way she was hoping. I asked this in as many ways as I could. Mostly she would shake her head and tell me 'But it will!'

We all felt quite helpless in the face of her steadfast conviction that she would be cured. We also doubted that she would even be well enough to go home for Peter's birthday party.

Thankfully, by Friday, the day before the party, Miriam's symptoms seemed well controlled and she even seemed a little stronger. David made arrangements to collect her before the party was due to start.

And with David's love and support and her determination, she made it. She returned in the evening happy but exhausted.

I hadn't been at work over the weekend but heard that she had been able to make the trip home.

On Monday I went in to see Miriam and was met by her beaming smile. David was with her and looked more relaxed than I had seen him in a while.

'You look happy,' I commented.

'Yes,' she said, 'I got a miracle!'

When Miriam was ready, her concept of what constituted a miracle for her had shifted.

This was again a lesson in just how important it is to patiently support a person in their reality and to be completely attentive. Simply, to be present. Their inner journeying will provide the necessary emotional and spiritual healing. Our, often impatient, agenda for them will not.

Chapter 4

FAMILIES

Palliative care commits to supporting the family/whānau as well as the patient. Families come in all sorts of shapes and sizes. It can be easy to make assumptions of the family group. And sometimes it is family members that need the most time and support. The following are two examples of different families' relationships, one damaging and one unconditionally loving.

Grief that damages

Graham

I walked into Graham's room in the hospital's palliative care inpatient unit. This was not going to be easy. I was about to meet Graham and Judy, a young couple who had just arrived. Graham was just 26 years old and Judy four years younger. They were recently engaged, with their whole lives ahead of them.

They did not belong here. They were far too young, weren't they?

Graham was a newly graduated accountant with a bright future. Judy, an outgoing and vivacious young woman, had been a receptionist at the accountancy firm where they had met. They were immediately attracted to one another. They adored each other.

But their lives had fallen apart.

Graham had malignant melanoma. He had secondaries in his liver and in his bones, causing awful pain. This had been difficult to manage at home and his gaunt face showed his suffering.

I sat down beside Graham's hospital bed. Judy was on the other side, with her head on Graham's shoulder.

Inwardly I took a deep breath. These two were not much older than my own children. How was I going to be able to ease their inevitable suffering? I knew that controlling Graham's physical symptoms would be relatively straight forward. But what of the emotional and existential suffering of these two young people?

They were in the palliative care unit's family/whānau room. This was a comfortably furnished room with a concertina door down the middle. This meant that it could be divided into two private single rooms if necessary. However, now it was one room with a hospital bed for Graham at one end. The other end of the room was furnished with comfortable chairs and had a fold down convertible couch. This allowed Judy to stay with him overnight. She was adamant that she was going to stay by his side.

When Graham was diagnosed with bone and liver secondaries, he and Judy had resigned their jobs and decided to move to be closer to his family; a decision he and Judy came to regret.

As well as the devastating diagnosis, his awful symptoms and the loss of their dreams together, the couple were faced with acrimony from Graham's parents.

I met Graham's parents the day after Graham was admitted. They were an imposing couple. His father was more than six foot three like his son, broad shouldered, with an almost military demeanour. Graham's mother was elegant and always immaculately dressed. They did not like Judy. They were prosperous dairy farmers and owned a beautiful large property. Judy was certainly not good enough for their only son and heir. They did not want her there and they certainly did not want her to be involved in his care.

Although Graham was 26 years old, his parents wanted to control all decisions made concerning his treatment and were nothing short of rude and nasty to Judy when she expressed an opinion.

Our role was to support Graham and his family, which to Graham very much included Judy. She was his soul mate. But Judy would often be found in tears after Graham's parents had visited.

'We're his parents,' they would say. 'We know what he needs. He needs rest. Not you mooning over him and upsetting him all the time.'

We knew that Graham's parents were hurting and grieving and feeling helpless at what was happening to their son. This just does not happen to your child. But as an adult, Graham wanted and needed to remain in control of treatment decisions and be able to decide for himself who he wanted and needed with him.

Graham's parents tried everything they could to shut Judy out. They were rude to her, telling her what damage she was doing to their son. They complained to the staff that she was upsetting their son.

However, Graham and Judy were devoted to each other and during his admission they decided to get married in the inpatient unit, knowing that he had just a few short weeks to live.

Graham's parents, of course, put as many obstacles in the way as they could. They demanded that this should not be allowed to happen.

'He's too sick to make rational decisions,' they said.

'You have to stop this,' they demanded of us.

But Graham and Judy were determined.

Graham was very frail at the wedding; Judy radiant but so sad. Judy's mother was able to be there to support her. Until then she had not been able to be physically present for her daughter, as she lived and worked hundreds of miles away.

The wedding went well despite the stony faces of Graham's parents.

Despite all, Graham and Judy were clearly happy that they were able to achieve this goal.

Graham died peacefully two short weeks later with Judy beside him, holding his hand.

Sadly, Judy continued to be the focus of cruelty from Graham's parents. She was locked out of the flat that she and Graham had shared and his possessions were taken by them.

Judy was already devastated by Graham's death. She was completely bewildered and further traumatised by this behaviour. Not surprisingly she became deeply depressed and her grieving unbearable.

One of the roles of a palliative care service is to provide bereavement support after death. Judy accepted this wholeheartedly. She would come into the palliative care department for visits to the bereavement counsellor.

One day I happened to meet her on one of her visits. We spoke for a few minutes and then she burst into tears. She showed me some ugly cuts on her arms. Through her tears she told me that she had done this herself. She agreed that I should talk to her General Practitioner with whom she had a really good relationship. Together, her GP and I persuaded her to be admitted to a psychiatric unit. Here she started the slow healing process over the next three weeks.

Then, over a period of many, many months with the love and support of her mother, close friends and healthcare professionals the old, outgoing Judy returned.

Two years after Graham's death, I heard that she was able to start her nursing training.

The bereavement team had also offered their support to Graham's parents. However, they made it clear they did not see this as necessary.

While being able to understand the heartbreak of Graham's parents — your child is not supposed to die before you — I found it very hard to remain compassionate when seeing the damage they were causing. Their grief was understandable but it was almost certainly other old issues, their "unfinished business", that was also being stirred and consequently affected Judy in such a damaging way.

To this day, I have wondered what more we could

have done as a team to get beyond their apparent self-important, arrogant façade. They had been offered the services of the counsellor in the team during Graham's admission but were adamant that they did not need such help. Could they have been approached in a different way? Could there have been a way to ameliorate their suffering, both for their sakes and to prevent their devastating attacks on Judy?

What is a life worth?

Darlene

'There's a 17-year-old girl we would like you to see ...'

Already my heart sank at the implications of a patient so young dying. Thoughts crowded in. The grief of the family at the prospect of one dying so young must be terrible. And what of the reactions of the staff caring for her?

'She has cerebral palsy and has had many admissions for aspiration pneumonia . . .'

'Poor kid — why don't they let her die?' my thoughts ran.

'She has a foster mother who has cared for her since

she was a year old and we have had conversations with her that there will be no attempts at CPR and she won't go to ICU.' 'Sounds straightforward then,' I found a part of me thinking. 'Well, she's a foster child and so there won't be the same emotional bond.' And then pulling myself up, 'What a judgement! — call yourself understanding and caring?'

Darlene was in a single cubicle in the ward alongside the emergency department of the hospital. She was lying in the bed on her side with her neck arched with obvious deformity. Her arms were contracted at the elbows, her legs at the knees. She had an oxygen mask covering most of her face. Her relief carer, Kylie, who had known Darlene for 7 years, was sitting beside the bed and holding one of Darlene's tiny deformed hands. She looked worried. Kylie had encouraged Darlene's foster mother, Ann, to go home for a shower and rest as she had been keeping vigil for 36 hours.

Darlene lay there fighting for her life; gurgling, almost drowning in her secretions and barely conscious.

'The kindest thing would be for this soul to slip away as soon as possible,' I thought.

The emergency team had told Ann and Kylie that

Darlene would almost certainly not survive this admission. 'But we have been here before,' they both said. It wasn't a statement of denial — just fact.

'In fact, she has been worse than this and survived,' they told us.

'How could they want that, when this poor kid cannot move herself; cannot talk; just lies there and is totally dependent,' my thoughts went on.

Then I felt ashamed. I didn't think I could have that degree of constant devotion and care — especially for a child who was not my flesh and blood. Suddenly I was searching my soul. I remembered someone once saying that a community can be judged on how it cares for its most vulnerable. And I had seen myself as a caring person. But this was a different level of caring and devotion I was seeing in front of me.

Darlene's pneumonia was treated with antibiotics. We provided advice on helping the symptoms; the gasping shortness of breath and restlessness while this was happening. And, she improved.

On the third day I went into the room and was greeted with a dazzling smile from Darlene. Ann and Kylie knew how this completely dependent scrap of humanity could bring value and meaning to a whole room just by her smile and dancing eyes.

Such a humbling experience. What value does human life have? Darlene's carers demonstrated how much more they understood than I of the value of vulnerable, dependent humanity.

Chapter 5

ASSUMPTIONS

How often we so easily make assumptions about people. Understanding cultural expression and rituals is important but I am constantly reminded of the danger in making generalisations and assumptions. Whatever one's ethnicity or culture, there is an underlying commonality of human emotions and needs. But each person is unique with their own individual expression of those needs and aspirations, both which require respect. There is also much that underlies expressions of suffering. It is easy to make assumptions about the causes. They can be quite wrong and lead to missed opportunities to ease existential pain.

Cultural assumptions

Lee

We squeezed into the tiny, smelly lift. It took us up to the fourth floor of a large apartment block in one of the poorer parts of Kuala Lumpur. I was in Kuala Lumpur visiting a hospice which is exclusively a home care service and serves a large part of this multicultural city. In the lift with me were the hospice nurse and doctor who were about to see one of their patients, Lee. There was a sad elderly looking man in the lift. We all got out together on the fourth floor and went towards the flat where Lee lived. The man was going towards the same door and we realised that this man must be Lee's father. He spoke no English but the nurse was Chinese and introduced us. We went in together.

There, in the living area of the flat, was a thin man lying on a folded down plastic deck chair. He did not look comfortable. The flat appeared to have just two rooms and Lee slept in the living area.

He was just 40 years old and his cancer had left him paraplegic. He was single, no longer able to work, and was now utterly dependent on his parents for everything.

Lil, the nurse, spoke Chinese, Malay and English and the hospice doctor, Sarah, who was European, spoke English and Malay. The patient spoke a little English but his parents none. Lil, Sarah and Lee engaged in a complex three language conversation.

Because he could not move his lower body, Lee had developed a bedsore. Lil asked him to lie down on his side and then took down his dressing. I stood there feeling a bit like a spare part. Mother was standing by looking worried and with knitted brow.

I noticed that there were faded family photographs on the wall above where Lee lay. I pointed to one which seemed to be her wedding photo and then gestured towards her and her husband. She nodded with a smile. And we engaged in a nonverbal, head nodding, head shaking, smiling conversation. She pointed out her son in the family photo and then pointed at him.

Then she saw the gaping sore on his back. Her face showed her horror. I had never seen a bedsore so large. Her eyes met mine and she collapsed into my arms in sobs. Two mothers sharing the sadness of something which should not be happening to a son. She clung to me in her sadness and I held her.

Before our visit, I had been told that this family didn't really express their emotions and that this was "very Chinese". I had also been told that "Chinese don't hug".

But here was a spontaneous and natural interaction.

I was reminded once again, of the danger of making generalisations about the emotional responses in relation to culture.

My experience working with many different cultural and ethnic groups is just how wrong generalisations can be. Cultural practices and rituals are very important, of course, but there is a need to approach each person as an individual with individual needs, views and values. We need to take each person's lead as to what is acceptable and appropriate.

Lee's mother needed and wanted to cry and be hugged.

My way: a peaceful death?

Ella

I did not recognise Ella when she came into the hospice inpatient unit. I had met her about a year before at a function that she had arranged to honour a visiting dignitary.

Ella was 49 years old and originally from South Korea but New Zealand was now her home. She was a recognised and respected leader of the Korean community where she lived; a mentor for many. Ella was known for her strong and forthright personality. She had a strong Buddhist faith that was incredibly important to her, as it was to her family too. She lived with her husband who was a complementary health practitioner.

Sadly, now, she needed admission to the hospice. Ella had a belly that was distended with tumour and most likely a bowel obstruction. One of my colleagues, who knew her well socially, expressed great relief that when Ella was offered an inpatient bed in the hospice she had accepted.

From the time of her diagnosis with advanced cancer Ella had remained very much in charge of her treatment, dictating exactly what cancer treatment and palliation she would or would not accept. Sometimes, for her friends and supporters and the healthcare professionals whom she would allow to advise her, this was somewhat difficult; in fact, sometimes a nightmare.

When she came into the hospice, she was in pain and suffered severe nausea and vomiting. The team felt confident they could control the worst of her symptoms and make her more comfortable. However, Ella and her husband continued to have very definite ideas about her management. And so, days of constant negotiation began. Some of the team became quite distressed that her symptoms remained less than well controlled.

'We're not doing our job properly,' they lamented.

'We should be controlling her symptoms so that she can die "peacefully".'

Her husband still believed strongly that she could be cured although it became clearer that Ella did not necessarily agree with him.

My colleague, her friend, made comment to us that Ella was preparing for the next part of her journey.

'She has always been like this,' he said. 'You can't tell her what to do.'

Some of her carers, however, had continued to find this hard to accept.

Ella did start to trust our advice more and did in fact even overrule her husband when he forbade us to give her some more morphine when her pain got worse.

Ella's daughter, a pharmacist, arrived from overseas and we thought that she would support the team's medication advice to her mother. How wrong we were. She wanted her mother to have intravenous supplements that we knew would not only be useless but could cause her mother's body to overload with fluid.

Ella chose to take the team's advice.

Gradually it became evident that Ella was deteriorating and that she would die within a few days. Her vomiting and pain were improved but certainly not controlled. The team did what they could and what was allowed.

Then in the middle of one night her vomiting became volcanic.

She died in a sea of vomit. The nurses looking after her that night were devastated and felt guilty that this could have happened. They believed that palliative care patients are supposed to die peacefully with their symptoms controlled.

But, how important it had been to accept and honour Ella's wishes and her need to control her own management. As healthcare professionals, our job was to support and advise her. It was her right and need to accept or reject that advice. It was up to us to deal with our sense of helplessness and judgement when our way was not her way.

A couple of mornings after Ella's death, one of the wonderful nurses who had cared for her the night she died met me with great excitement and disbelief. Ella's death notice was in the morning paper. It described how she had died *very peacefully*. The team was also thanked for all the wonderful care that she had received. Perception is everything.

It may have been that Ella's family did see a peacefulness for Ella in how her last days and moments unfolded. Or perhaps their culture obliged them to say that. We will never know for sure but Ella had done it her way. And it was us who were distressed because it wasn't the way we thought it should be.

Assumptions about suffering

James

James looked uncomfortable and miserable. He was sitting in a La-Z-Boy leaning forward with his chest heaving. He was in the hospice inpatient unit and his nurse, May, and I had just walked into the room. May introduced me to him as this was the first time I had met James. He looked up at me imploringly.

'You look really uncomfortable,' I said. 'Let's get you some pain relief.'

'My chest hurts so much and I can't breathe properly.'

While the nurse went to get pain relief, I sat down beside James.

'Where in your chest does it hurt?' I asked.

'Where they did that talc thing!' he said and burst into tears. He was distraught.

Once he had had some pain relief, May and I sat quietly with him. His sobs settled but he looked exhausted. He closed his eyes.

'We'll come back a bit later to talk if that's ok,' I said. James nodded.

As we left, May said to me, 'The talc pleurodesis was so awful that the pain is all he can think about. It always upsets him. And he's such an anxious man.'

James was 60 years old and had secondary cancer in his lungs. He had been admitted to the inpatient hospice unit with uncontrolled pain. He had a long history of anxiety and an apparent sensitivity to pain medications. This had made his pain management difficult. He also had developed fluid around his lung which kept coming back. About two weeks previously he had been admitted to hospital for the fluid to be drained from the pleural space. Talc had been inserted between the two layers of pleura to try and stick them together and prevent the fluid recurring. This is often a painful procedure if pain management is not well attended to. Where the drain had been removed was the site of his worst pain.

When I met James, he had been in the inpatient unit for a few days. His pain had improved but control was not optimal. I hoped more could be done.

As we had promised, May and I went back to see James that afternoon. His wife Pat was with him now. She held his hand and seemed to have a calming influence on him. We talked about his pain medications and previous difficulties with some. As soon as the "talc thing" was mentioned he again became really upset and sobbed. He looked really scared. Pat shook her head as she said, 'It was really horrible for him.'

That evening I thought about James, his distressed response and his obvious anxiety. I wondered whether he would be open to acupoint tapping. This includes a number of techniques which include tapping on the upper body acupressure points. It is useful for working with emotional distress and was first shown to be particularly helpful for anxiety and phobias. The techniques will be described later. The one I use is simple, easily learnt and can be introduced as a relaxation technique.

The next morning, I offered to teach James and he was very keen. Pat was particularly enthusiastic and encouraged him. As we tapped together, he became visibly more relaxed and his breathing became freer. When he talked about the talc experience he again become upset. As we talked and tapped, it became clear that it wasn't the actual pain that haunted him. Rather he was distressed that the doctor who had done the procedure and the assisting nurse had barely acknowledged him. They left without speaking to him and apparently without concern for him.

One of the tapping interventions recently developed by Steve Wells, psychologist, focusses on the meaning that attaches to an event or issue. For James that attachment was about being disregarded and a sense of abandonment rather than the actual physical pain of the procedure. Using Intention Tapping, as Steve has called it, James visibly relaxed and even smiled. After fifteen to twenty minutes, however, he was very tired and so I left him. I suggested that he use the tapping points whenever his anxiety was troubling him.

The next day the staff reported that when the talc pleurodesis was mentioned or referred to he no longer became distressed. Importantly, this lack of emotional response was sustained in coming days.

When I saw James a couple of days later he appeared more frail, was coughing and nauseated. He looked anxious and miserable.

'I think he's only got a few days,' said the nurse. James certainly looked as if that might be true.

I sat beside him. 'How are you doing?' I said.

'Not great,' he replied. With tears in his eyes, he continued. 'My son doesn't even know I've got cancer, let alone that I might die soon. He lives in Germany. I know I should call him but I'm too scared. He might try and come back to New Zealand and he can't because he's in the Military Police there.'

I must have looked a little puzzled because James went on to explain that he hadn't really been part of his son Martin's growing up.

'I split up from his mother when he was a toddler and she took him to live in Germany. I really regret not having seen him for so many years. But I went to Germany about three years ago. We got on like a house on fire. I'm so proud of him! He's in the Military Police and doing really well. But I haven't seen him for two years.' All of this came tumbling out. It exhausted him and he fell back on the pillows. I suggested that we do some more tapping on his anxiety and he nodded. He was tired and so I asked his permission to tap on the points for him. Ten minutes was the limit of James' energy but just these few minutes calmed him.

I was not working in the unit for the next couple of weeks but heard that James' condition deteriorated and his symptoms of nausea, cough and anxiety worsened over a few days. The staff assumed he was very close to dying and his symptoms were treated, with emphasis on medications. However, one of my colleagues who is also proficient in tapping techniques became involved in James' care. She identified that his main suffering was that he still had not spoken to his son, Martin.

Using Intention Tapping again, she worked with James around his anxiety and why he remained worried about phoning his son.

That night James spoke to Martin. The conversation went well, with lots of tears but lots of healing. The next day, James was more relaxed, and appeared more physically comfortable. About a week later, his symptoms were controlled sufficiently for him to go home. He died peacefully and pain-free at home two weeks later with Pat by his side.

James' story reinforced for me how important it is to not make assumptions about what peoples' symptoms and emotional responses are about and what they represent. We need to look deeper. It also emphasised the value and strength of working in a team able to provide consistency of approach.

Chapter 6

ACCEPTANCE

When someone looks or behaves differently it is easy to judge them. Can I see beyond the behaviour and what it implies of that person? How do I accept the person but not the behaviour? Mark and his interactions with hospice staff taught me about the power of acceptance.

The power of acceptance

Mark

We were met outside by a prison guard. He unlocked the first door electronically and led us inside to a small uninviting room. Here the guard examined our bags and then waved a wand over our bodies. The guard then smiled and the next door was unlocked. He then led us through a series of corridors and doors to the prison sickbay.

I was visiting the local prison with Mary, one of the hospice community nursing team.

We were there to visit an inmate, Mark, a man in his 40s who did not have long to live. He had advanced liver cancer diagnosed during his imprisonment and his pain was poorly controlled.

Mark had been a wanderer for most of his adult life, a seaman for a time and had certainly never had a place to call home. He had had many brushes with the law. Homelessness he knew well. He had been asleep under a tree one night when a police officer tried to wake him. Instinctively Mark had taken out his knife. He was convicted of threatening a police officer with a knife and hence landed up in prison for quite a stretch. His prison sentence had actually finished six weeks ago but there seemed to be nowhere that he could be released to.

Mary and I met with Mark at the prison together with the prison doctor. Mark was tall and skinny with long greasy, straggly hair and a patch over one eye. He had lost his eye in a knife fight in prison. He looked like an out of work pirate. The f-word and the s-word punctuated his speech. His manner was aggressive and very wary.

He glared at us. 'Who are these fucking people?'

The prison doctor glared at Mark. 'This is Dr Sue and Mary from the hospice. They've come to help you, so watch your language.'

Mark was clearly in physical pain, due to gross enlargement of the cancer in his liver. In prison the best form of pain relief had been deemed to be fentanyl patches. The trouble was these kept getting stolen.

How could we help?

Could we put aside our judgements and assumptions to provide the care and attention that he desperately needed?

'Can you take him into the hospice inpatient unit to control his symptoms and to allow him end of life care?' the prison doctor asked. I hesitated. Had we seen him in the community at large, I would have recommended he be admitted to the inpatient hospice unit. But, would this man be a danger to the hospice staff and the rest of the patients? Would he take our medication advice anyway? What sort of disruption would he cause?

This was something that needed to be discussed with the whole team. And so, we made some interim suggestions about pain management — and ways to secure his fentanyl patches — and went back to the hospice to discuss the situation.

We held a meeting and everyone spoke openly about the risks, their fears and judgements. How would this be for them and for the other patients? There was a free bed and the hospice had all single rooms with ensuite facilities.

We decided that Mark could be admitted as long as there was a personal security guard to protect the staff and other patients.

And so, Mark came to the inpatient unit. His room was bright and cheerful and comfortable. It was probably the most pleasant he had ever known. How dare he not be grateful. But the foul, aggressive and demanding language reflected anything but gratitude. When nurses went to attend to Mark, he rewarded them with a deluge of bad language. This had been Mark's means of communication for such a long time. We did realise that it was likely a front, covering a mass of fear, loneliness and grief, but that didn't make it acceptable.

The Nursing Director, Sally, wasn't going to put up with it. She looked at Mark and set the rules and boundaries.

'If you swear at the nurses like that and yell at them they will not come into your room!' Would Mark comply?

Later that day, Mark was in pain and pushed his call bell to request some pain relief. His allocated nurse arrived at the door.

'Took your fucking time!'

The nurse, without a word, turned and walked away.

Mark's mouth dropped open and he called after her.

'I'm sorry,' he said,' I didn't mean it.'

The nurse turned back and asked Mark what he needed.

'What the fuck do you think I need?'

Again, she turned and walked away.

'Oh, shit,' she heard him say. 'Please come back. The pain's killing me. I'm sorry,' he called out.

'Ok, Mark. I'll go and get some pain relief. I will be back with it as soon as I can.'

That night there was a similar exchange but that was the last of Mark's abuse towards the nurses.

Some time into his stay, Sally offered to take Mark to

the local shops in her car. When they got to the shops he was about to get out when he looked at Sally with alarm.

'I've had an accident and wet your seat!' Sally gulped and tried to reassure him.

'It's ok. I'm just joking!' he said, with a cheeky grin on his face.

Sally's face fell into her hands in great relief.

Mark went and did his shopping and when he returned, he presented Sally with a red rose.

Love can be seen as having two dimensions. Firstly, I accept who you are but not your behaviour. And secondly, your behaviour needs to have clear boundaries so that you don't hurt yourself and you don't hurt other people. So said that very wise woman, Elisabeth Kübler-Ross.

The change in Mark's behaviour once he was pain free and felt safe and accepted was remarkable.

Within a week, the team felt safe enough for themselves and for the other patients and their families to dispense with the security guard. Being able to accept another person but not their behaviour is such a thing of power and beauty.

Chapter 7

DIGNITY

'How can we help our dying rabies patients?' one of the doctors asked.

My mouth dropped open.

'What did you say?' I replied. Had I heard correctly?

At the time, I was visiting the Philippines about three times a year with two colleagues. We were there to help in the development of a palliative care programme in Manila at the Infectious Diseases Hospital. This hospital served the poor of Manila and the surrounding provinces. My professional background was in oncology before moving into palliative medicine. I had some experience in the palliation of non-malignant disease and a little in

AIDS. But rabies? I'd never seen a patient with rabies before.

However, the staff were asking me about care of these patients.

'Tell me about these patients,' I said once I had gathered my thoughts.

At the time, apparently some two patients a week were dying horrific deaths with rabies at the hospital. The patients were often young people and children. The staff described how a patient would present to the emergency department with typical symptoms including hydrophobia (fear of water), and within 72 hours they would die agitated, hallucinating and aggressive.

These patients clearly needed palliation. But how? When in doubt, back to basics. First identify the symptom complex. This was clearly an agitated delirium which should respond to anti-psychotic medications, for example haloperidol. Haloperidol is relatively cheap and was usually available at the hospital. The availability of medications was a constant difficulty for this fledgling palliative care group.

Identifying what needed to be done for these patients was only part of the problem. Persuading staff that they might be able to be palliated was another huge hurdle. 'Nothing will work', we were told. Changing practices often happens very slowly. It in fact took nearly two years before haloperidol became established for use in rabies delirium at the hospital.

Final requests and dignity

Jojo

My first rabies patient was Jojo.

We had just arrived for one of our visits to the hospital.

'A rabies patient has just been admitted,' my Filipino colleague, Ceri, exclaimed.

'Will you come and see him? We have some haloperidol available for him.' Ceri was excited as they had only used haloperidol once before for a rabies patient.

Jojo was 25 years old. He had come to the hospital from a rural area and was diagnosed with the early symptoms of rabies. He knew that with the diagnosis came a death sentence and that he had just hours or days to live. He knew that his dying would be with the worst suffering he could imagine, that he would behave like a rabid dog, foaming at the mouth and die in agony. He also knew that he would be alone in a locked cell tied to a bed, as he would be seen as dangerous. His saliva would be infectious and so staff and family would have to keep away in case he bit them or spat at them, especially in their eyes. This was how rabies patients had been managed up until now as it was believed that nothing could control their symptoms.

It was thus that I met Jojo. The room was a bleak cell. The only window was tiny, high and barred. The door was barred with a large lock. Jojo was tied to a bed by his ankles and wrists to await his fate.

I stood there for a minute with Ceri and looked. I tried to smile at Jojo.

Then his young, very pregnant wife, Maria, walked in. She was 19 years old and pregnant with their second child. She spoke no English and despite what was happening to her husband smiled broadly at me and then shook her head sadly. She then sat down on the bench across from her husband and started to eat the food she had just brought in. It all seemed surreal. My feelings were completely jumbled. Here was a desperate situation — JoJo would surely be dead in 72 hours. Yet there was a calmness and an acceptance in the young couple. Or perhaps they didn't know what was going to happen?

The breadwinner of this poor young family was about to die. I couldn't take it in. Ceri asked me if I would like to take a photo. It seemed to me such an intrusion and quite wrong. However, she assured me it would be perfectly fine to ask. Jojo and his wife seemed almost delighted to be asked and Maria sat up with her huge smile while I took a photo. This photo has become very precious to me.

I wondered whether Jojo really did understand what was happening.

However, at this point, he looked up at me and said with pleading eyes, 'Please don't let me suffer.'

We were just starting the protocol using regular haloperidol to try and control the agitated delirium and had some available. My eyes met his and I felt inadequate.

All I could say was, 'I promise we will try our best.'

His next plea came.

'Can I see my daughter before I die?' His daughter was just two years old.

Two simple requests. I hoped we could make them happen. Yes, we could.

The haloperidol protocol worked. By controlling his symptoms his two final requests could be fulfilled. His little daughter was allowed to visit and 48 hours later Jojo died calmly and peacefully.

Dealing with unfinished business

Orlando

Orlando lay there tied to the bed. He was a man in his 40s, with a wife and four teenage children. He had lots to live for but was dying of rabies. Rabies. He would be dead 54 hours from diagnosis. He knew that people who die from rabies have excruciating deaths, like rabid dogs.

He looked at me with dark anguished eyes and asked, 'Is this a punishment from God? Will I go to heaven?' A deeply religious man, he was asking *me*, a non-Catholic, non-Christian questions about his soul's future.

We had recently started using haloperidol to control the agitated delirium that rabies patients suffer at the end of their lives.

We were planning to commence it for Orlando as soon as he was diagnosed and admitted. However, when Orlando was diagnosed there was no haloperidol available in the hospital nor surrounding pharmacies. What could we do? Again, we needed to resort to first principles. In this case — use whatever you have and use it regularly. We therefore opted to use high doses of regular diazepam intramuscularly. This would be painful and not ideal but what was the alternative?

So far Orlando had remained calm and lucid with the alternate regimen. Hence we were able to at least have a little time to address the less physical aspects of his suffering.

However, knowing our medication management was less than ideal, this added another level to *my* anxiety of trying to address the struggle facing this man's soul. I was the only one in the room and the priest was not available. I knew that I must respond to his haunting question. He needed my heart to talk to his heart, my soul to his.

'Orlando, I don't believe this is a punishment from God,' I said. 'And I believe that you will be in your heaven. But tell me, why do you think this might be a punishment from God?'

Tearfully he said, 'I had an affair and my wife doesn't know about it. It was before I met Maria but I feel so guilty.'

I had to try hard to put to one side my feelings about a religion that sometimes engendered guilt that could lead a man to torture himself like this.

'Perhaps, Orlando, you could ask her,' I suggested.

He looked doubtful but agreed that he would like to try. The medication was preventing the dangerous raging delirium which would have previously prevented contact with anyone. I found his wife and we sat with Orlando.

He sheepishly told her how guilty he felt and asked if she could forgive him.

Maria looked at him and gave a little laugh.

'It was before we met. It doesn't matter at all!'

Orlando's whole body visibly relaxed. His eyes filled with tears of gratitude as he looked at her.

Next he asked about his four children. Could he see them? His wife and the nursing staff gasped at the thought. Would it be safe? However, Orlando was still calm, still lucid and still having painful two hourly loadings with diazepam.

The children aged between 16 and 12 years old came into the room and shyly stood beside their dad. He told them how much he loved them and that because he had rabies he would surely die very soon.

It was one of the most poignant moments I have ever witnessed.

Twenty-four hours later, Orlando died peacefully.

These two men taught me so much about the critical importance of the basic principles of palliative care. Excellent symptom management can be achieved with extremely limited resources. This, in turn, can allow attention to be focussed on emotional and existential suffering. As such, there is a higher possibility of at least a degree of peace at the end of life.

Chapter 8

IMAGES OF THE SOUL

(symbolic language, the language of spirituality and impromptu drawings)

As Aristotle said, 'The soul never thinks without an image.'

I was first introduced to the use of impromptu drawings as a communication tool by Elisabeth and her team. Later, I had the good fortune to meet and learn from Gregg Furth, a Jungian psychologist from New York. He had managed to expand this technique into the realm of everyday therapy.

Essentially, the client is given a simple box of crayons and a piece of paper and invited to draw an image of what they are feeling or what it is they are trying to express.

I came to find the use of impromptu drawings helpful in:

1. Enhancing communication, i.e. by helping to start a dialogue
2. To help ventilate feelings, i.e. externalisation
3. To help bring information into consciousness using symbolic images.

Impromptu drawings seem to be the symbolic language coming from the spiritual aspect of the artist. Elisabeth said that symbolism is the language of spirituality.

Certainly this seemed to be the case for Leonie, Eddie and Arran, the people I would like to tell you about.

Journeying with pictures

Leonie

I had known Leonie for several months when she came into the palliative care clinic one day. She had been severely short of breath from lung secondaries and this had been really difficult to manage. Today her breathing was not really troubling her. But something was. She looked different, solemn and bemused.

'I've hit an emotional and spiritual wall,' she said.

What did she mean?

Leonie was just 42 years old and the mother of three energetic teenagers. She had metastatic bowel cancer with lung and liver secondaries. At about the time of her diagnosis her husband had left her for one of her friends. Fortunately, she had wonderfully supportive siblings and came from a large Roman Catholic family with a very strong faith.

I was curious.

'Can you explain a bit more about what you mean by an emotional and spiritual wall?' I asked. 'You look different.'

'I don't know what to say,' she said. She sounded frustrated and a little agitated.

Words were not going to help and so I asked her to draw a picture.

The picture she drew follows.

I thought it looked chaotic and confusing but I knew that I should not try and interpret what she had drawn.

'Can you tell me about your drawing?' I asked.

'That's my coffin,' she said. 'It all feels so confusing and scary.'

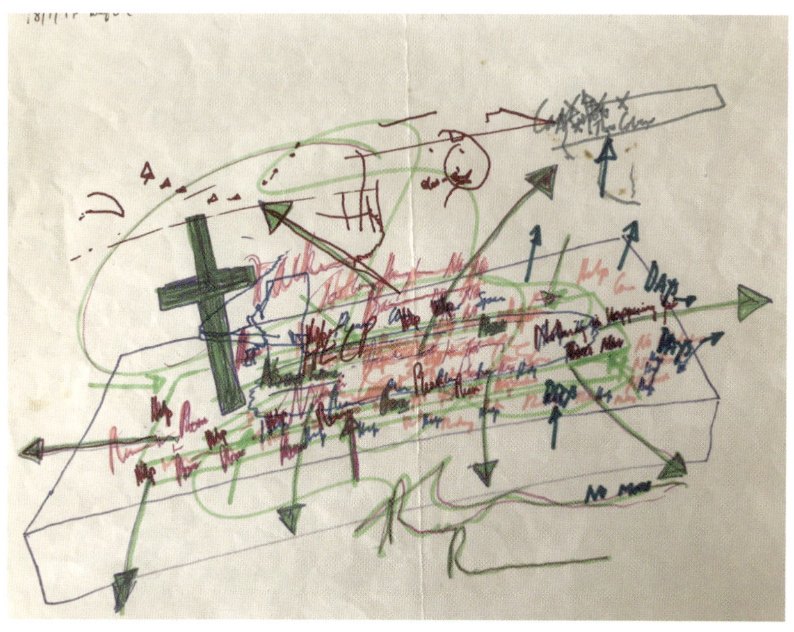

I drew her attention to the arrows going into and out of the coffin. 'Can you tell me about those?' I asked.

'Those are my thoughts,' she said. 'Sometimes I think about what it's going to be like and those squiggles are my messed-up thoughts. And sometimes it all seems clear,' she said, pointing to the longer arrows coming from the coffin. 'It feels like that's what is happening in my body.'

As we talked, focussing our attention on the picture she had drawn she became less withdrawn and a little more her usual cheerful self.

A few days later I visited her at home. Her thoughts appeared to be far away.

'I feel kind of weird,' she said. 'I can't really describe it.'

Again I asked her to draw a picture and this is what she drew.

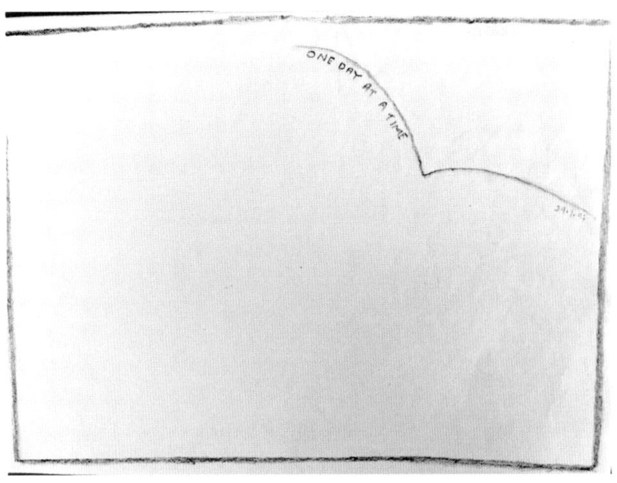

She looked at her picture and said, 'It's like I am a seagull circling over the world and I'm not in my body. I just have to take one day at a time.' She looked puzzled. Then she drew some more pictures.

I asked her about the squares that she had drawn. 'That's my bed quilt,' she said. 'That's me in the square,' she said, pointing to the seagull image she had drawn.

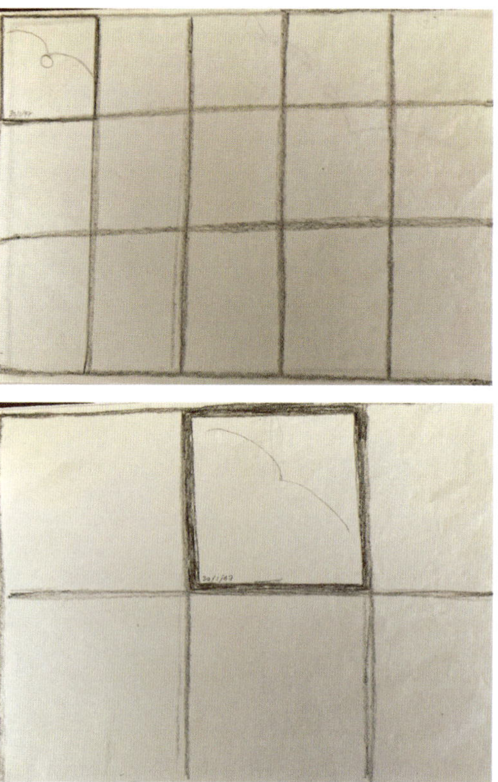

I suggested that she might like to do further drawings over the next few days to see what might happen. Gradually, the seagull seemed to have more of a body and, gradually, even some colour.

And the sequence certainly coincided with Leonie becoming seemingly more present in her body and more of her bubbly self. And of this picture she stated emphatically, 'I'm more focussed.'

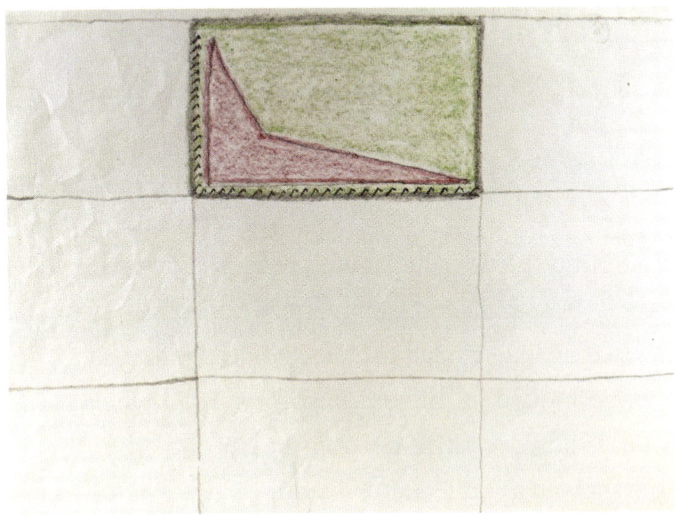

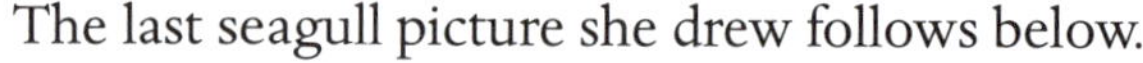

The last seagull picture she drew follows below.

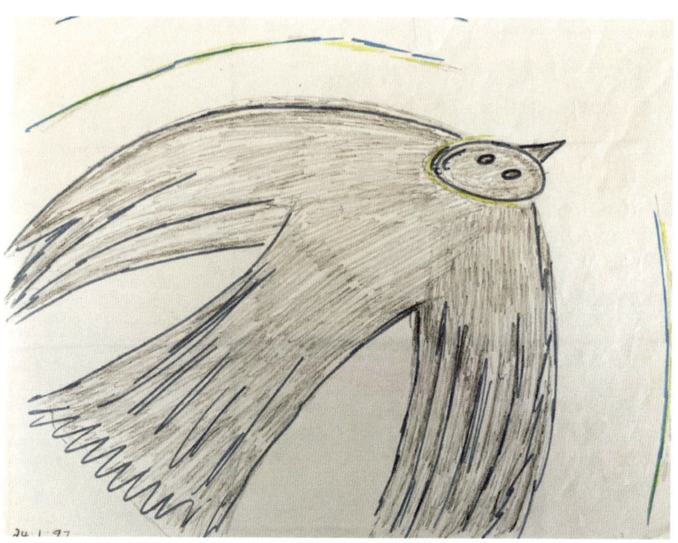

Intrigued I asked her about the seagull that seemed to have its head pulled in with no neck. I asked her whether the seagull had needed to "keep its head pulled in".

She looked at me and said, 'Yes, I did when I was little. I didn't want to get abused like the others.' Her face showed a sudden understanding. This led to Leonie and her sisters later talking about the verbal abuse and occasional corporal punishment that had occurred when they were young. They had never discussed this before.

The last picture Leonie drew four weeks before she died was so very different from her first.

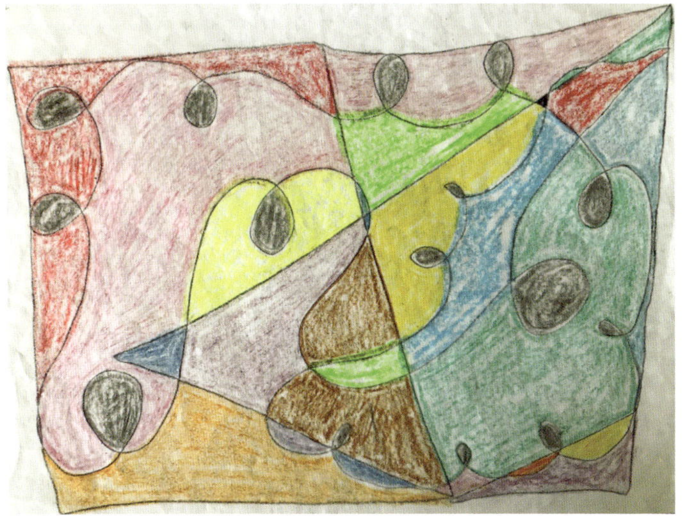

'Tell me about this one,' I said. 'It looks a little different to the first picture you drew.'

She described how much more peaceful she was now feeling.

'I know I am going to die. I'm sad but somehow it's ok.'

'What are the grey spots about?' I asked.

She looked at me wistfully. 'Those are the pockets of grief about leaving my kids.'

As Leonie became frailer and more confined to home, she was cared for by her two sisters who were both nurses, one of them a very experienced palliative care nurse.

One day I arrived at the door and was greeted by the sisters who were laughing. 'She's talking about potatoes and poker machines!'

As a family they had all travelled a long way in accepting Leonie's cancer and knew that she would die soon. They were an inspirational family; pragmatic, caring, with a faith that supported them. They also all had a wonderful sense of humour. From their description when I arrived at the door, I wondered if Leonie may have developed a delirium.

I went to her room and she greeted me as usual.

I sat on her bed and asked her how she was. As we talked, she didn't seem to have disordered thought. So, I asked her, 'What's this about potatoes and poker machines?' She gave a slightly exasperated laugh. 'I have had this image of one of those sort of poker machines or do you call them fruit machines? It's one of those things where you have to somehow get a match of three fruits in a row. In this case I was trying to get three potatoes in a row.' She looked frustrated.

'Well, what do potatoes mean to you?' I asked.

She immediately responded, 'Nutrition! Sustenance!'

Remembering her strong Catholic faith, somehow it occurred to me that the three potatoes might have something to do with the Trinity.

'Mmm … nutrition and sustenance,' I repeated. 'If that's what they mean, what do you think it would take to get the potatoes in a row?'

She looked pensive and then she smiled. 'I just need to open my heart and let the Holy Spirit in — that's the third potato!' and then she relaxed onto her pillows.

Leonie died peacefully just 48 hours later.

Dreams

Eddie

I first met Eddie when he was admitted to the hospital inpatient unit. His lung cancer had come back, causing pain and shortness of breath.

My first impression of him was that he was a fastidious, somewhat boring elderly gentleman. His symptoms were improving but he looked sad and rather apathetic. His wife of 40 years had died three months before and the team assumed he was deeply grieving.

I went in to see him one morning and sat down. I asked him how his night had been. He gave me a curious look and said, 'Well, I had a weird dream. I dreamt about my house and all the rooms were dark except one, which was light and bright.'

'That sounds interesting,' I responded. 'Do you have any idea what it's about?'

'It's my house and where I lived with my wife. You know she died? But I really don't know what it's about.'

'I did know that your wife died. I am sorry.' We sat for a moment and then I said 'I wonder, Eddie, if you could draw the house?'

Drawing a representation of a dream was part of Gregg Furth's teaching. It could help to make sense of what the subconscious is trying to tell us.

'Don't be silly!' said Eddie. 'I can't draw.'

'I'm not suggesting a masterpiece Eddie, perhaps just an outline of the house and its rooms?' I smiled at him.

'Ok,' he said. 'I'll give it a go. I haven't much else to do!' I went and got some paper and crayons before he changed his mind.

Later that day I went back and was surprised to see that he had drawn two pictures.

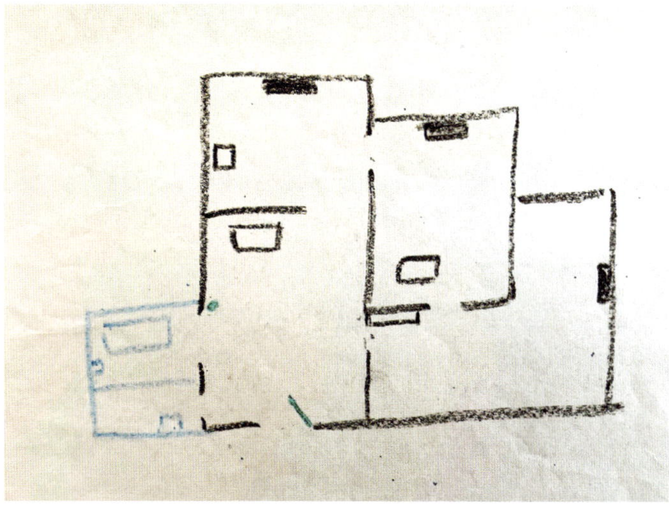

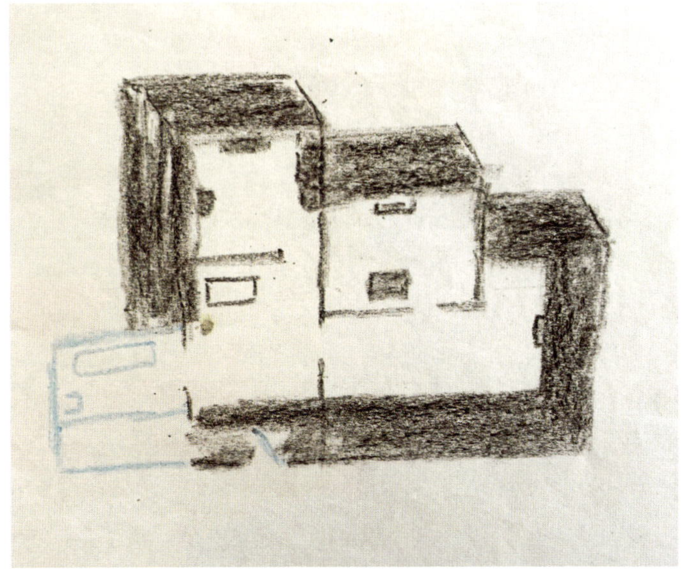

'I drew out the plan as you told me to.' I wasn't sure that I had been quite so directive but it became clear that he was used to doing what he was instructed. 'Then I thought I wanted to put thicker walls around most of the rooms like in my dream.'

'Can you say more about that, and the room you have drawn in blue?'

'The blue room is where all the washing and cleaning happens. The other rooms are the bedrooms and lounge and my wife's sewing room.'

'I notice one of the rooms has a smaller door than the others.' He looked at me, then at the picture, and then back at me.

'The room with the narrow door is my wife's sewing room. I was never allowed in there,' he said with a sigh. 'You'll probably think I'm awful and don't get me wrong. I am sad she died. But it always felt as if she squashed anything I wanted to do. I used to be quite creative you know. It's almost like the "washing" room is like my escape and now I can be more creative again.' All this came tumbling out. He looked surprised at himself.

Eddie gave me those first pictures. I showed them to a young colleague and asked what he thought, knowing Eddie's cancer history. 'Well,' he said. 'It looks as if everything has been black since his wife died and his cancer recurred. I think he sees that he is going to die soon. The blue room represents his death and escape from this life and he wants to join his wife.' His mouth dropped open when I told him how Eddie had described his drawing. My colleague had fallen into the trap of putting *his* interpretation onto the drawing.

Eddie went home from the unit soon after that. He would come to the outpatient clinic regularly. Each time he came he brought a new picture with him. They were more and more colourful. He drew pictures of his garden and how he had laid it out. There were beautiful spring flowers and lush shrubs. Sometimes he would bring in a bunch of his blooms. He had discovered his creativity.

One day when he came to the clinic he looked pensive. 'What's up, Eddie?' I enquired.

'Had another strange dream last night. I dreamt a panther was chasing me.'

'Goodness. That sounds dramatic. What happened?'

'Oh, I shot it,' he said. This seemed like a very important dream and so again I suggested he draw it. 'OK' he said, 'I think I will. It was very vivid.'

The next time I saw Eddie he showed me these masterpieces.

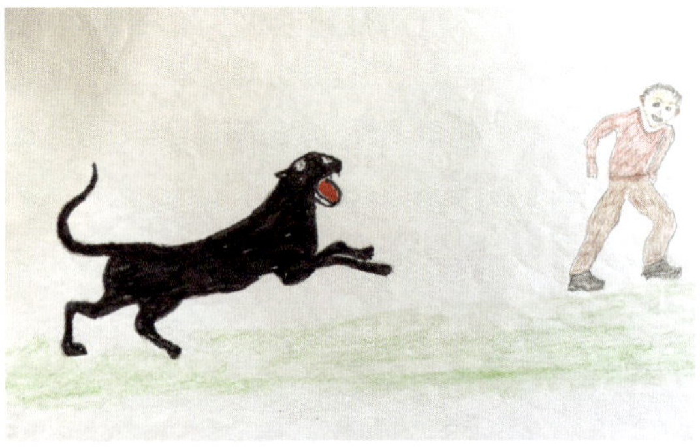

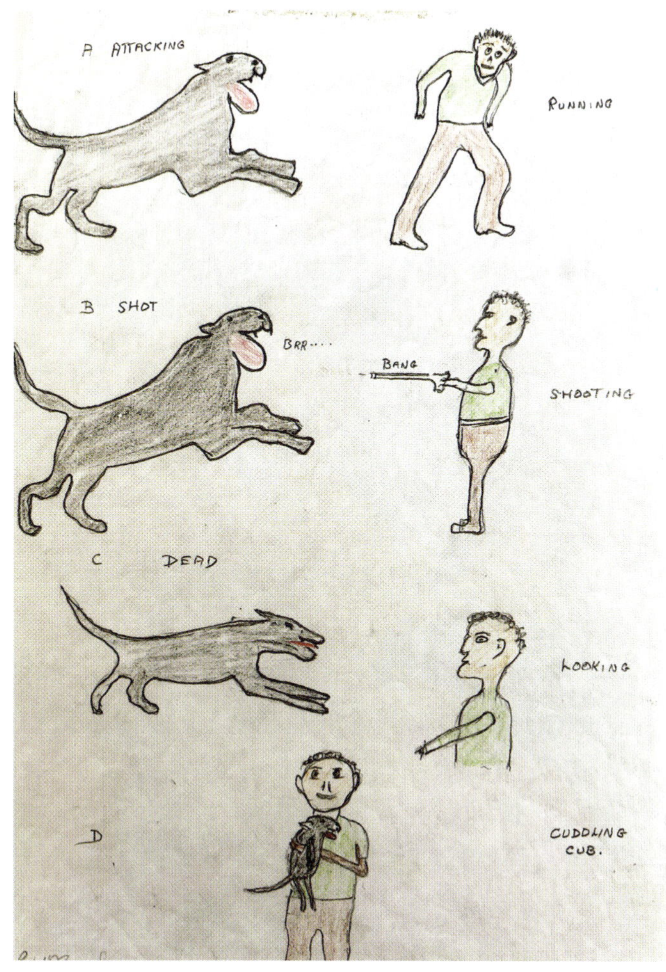
A ATTACKING
RUNNING
B SHOT
BRR....
BANG
SHOOTING
C DEAD
LOOKING
D
CUDDLING
CUB.

'Wow!' I said, 'You've become quite an artist. Tell me about this panther!'

'Well, the panther is my cancer, of course! I had that special treatment last year if you remember. So that's shooting the cancer and killing it. I've written down what I think it means. The cancer has come back.'

I looked at him and nodded.

'But you know, I'm interested in the look on your face in the series you've drawn. Look at the first and the last.'

He grinned at me. 'I was so scared when I was first diagnosed last year. Now I know it's grown back but I'm not scared. It's almost as if I've made friends with the new cub!!'

Eddie continued to nurture his garden, growing all sorts of plants. Orchids became his passion in his conservatory as he became less able to garden outside. Eventually the new cub grew into an adult.

This delightful man taught me a lot about the danger of assumptions. And, he embraced the wonderful possibility of growth and creativity, even towards the end of life.

My interpretation of the Panther drawings
when related to my illness.

'reviously I had been told I had cancer +
was coping well.

X indicates

The cancer tumour grew rapidly.
I was told that I had, no hope only
about three weeks to live

I had to repel it so I shot it.
The only thing I could do was accept spear
treatment which would destroy the tumour

This treatment apparently killed the
growth + for 15 months the cancer
has been dormant.

Holding a new cub.

This indicates a restart of the cancer

Inner knowledge

Alan

Alan was one of the first patients referred to the palliative care team at the regional tertiary hospital. Although each team member was an experienced clinician, coming together as this team was new. Supporting Alan and his family challenged each of us not just clinically but also in how the team functioned and related to other services.

Alan was just 25 years old, a lively young man with a wonderful future.

Why does such a young man come to be dying of cancer? And he had malignant melanoma — one of the cruellest.

Alan had had a skin melanoma removed in his teens. Unfortunately, the melanoma reared its ugly head again in his twenties and spread. His brain became involved. This was treated with surgery and radiotherapy but by now he also had bone secondaries. And so he was referred to the palliative care service for symptom management and any support that the team could give him and his family.

Alan was the youngest in the family with three older sisters. They were a pragmatic farming family. Our job was to support and accept where Alan and each of his family members were on this lonely grief journey.

Some of the team felt that Alan's father was distant and uninvolved. But this man was grieving and hurting so much. His only son was to be taken from him. Where was our compassion when judging this man's responses and ways of getting through this tragedy? Each person's experience of the same event is personal, unique and is often very lonely despite the closeness of others.

And yes, Alan himself challenged the team over several months when we saw him regularly as an outpatient. Sometimes he would turn up unannounced demanding to see one of the team. He had painful bone secondaries for which he received radiotherapy with a good response but he continued to need ongoing medications. Sometimes other symptoms were bothering him. Sometimes his medications had run out and he had forgotten to fill his prescriptions. Sometimes he had muddled up his forms for his welfare payments. Sometimes he just wanted to chat and hang out. Which services was the team best able to provide and which were better provided by others?

Well, Alan challenged all of this. As a young man, what did any of the rules that health services tend to make mean to him? Also, because of his brain secondaries he had difficulty at times with his memory and thought processes.

As the months went by, it became clear that Alan was becoming frailer and sicker. The disease had involved his bone marrow and so from time to time he was admitted for transfusions and the improvement of his symptom management.

During one of his admissions, when I was sitting talking to Alan, it was clear that he was having difficulty expressing what was on his mind and in his heart.

I suggested that he draw a picture.

This is what Alan drew.

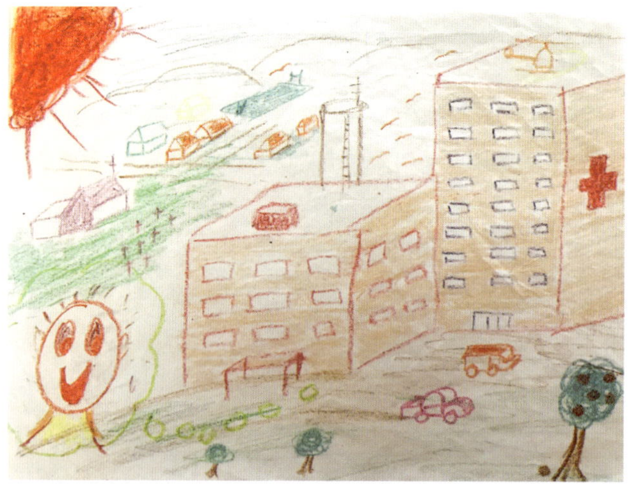

Alan's picture reminded me of a technique that Elisabeth used when looking at impromptu drawings where each quadrant of the page represents a period of time.[1]

Together Alan and I explored his drawing. One should never *interpret* what another has drawn but merely ask questions. Only the artist knows what is represented. He talked about being in hospital, and pointed to the building he had clearly drawn centrally and in the top right quadrant of the picture. He talked about what it was like for him to be in hospital and not be able to do the things other people his age were doing. It started a conversation about his lost dreams for his future. 'I can't do what my friends are doing. They are going out and having fun. They have jobs. They're getting married ...' There were tears in his eyes and he was clearly angry at the unfairness.

I asked about the smiling face in the bottom left corner.

'That's me when I was happy at home doing stuff on the farm,' he said wistfully. 'I can't do any of those things anymore.'

'And what is going on here?' I said, pointing to the tree

in the bottom right corner. 'There seems to be five apples on the tree and one on the ground.'

'That's my family,' he said, again with tears in his eyes. 'Those are my parents and sisters on the tree. I am about to drop off.' He pointed to the apple on the ground. This was the first time I had heard him refer to his death.

And what about the buildings and what appeared to be the sun that he had drawn in the remaining quadrant of the page? Alan confirmed that he had drawn a very orange sun. 'I used to love the sun and being outside,' he said. He then described the little town he had grown up in. There was the school with the rugby field, the houses and the church. He pointed to the crosses beside the church and without any further prompting said, 'That's where I am going to be buried soon.' There was a mixture of sadness and anger in his voice. He started to become really angry.

Elisabeth once said that when a person draws a sun in the top left quadrant of an impromptu drawing the artist is not afraid of death. I have never been completely sure of this, but that was Elisabeth's experience and she had explored thousands of drawings with their artists. Interestingly, I didn't have the sense that Alan was scared of death. But I got the real sense that he was furious about the fact that he would die soon. This seemed to be expressed in the intensity of his colouring of the sun in his picture. It was almost as if he had ground the colour into it.

Yes, Alan was angry and I got the sense he would really have loved to release some of that emotion physically; perhaps even with a punching bag or even just running and shouting. However, his physical condition did not even really allow him to go for a decent walk. I suggested to Alan that he could perhaps put his anger into a picture.

He needed to externalise these feelings somehow.

This is what he drew.

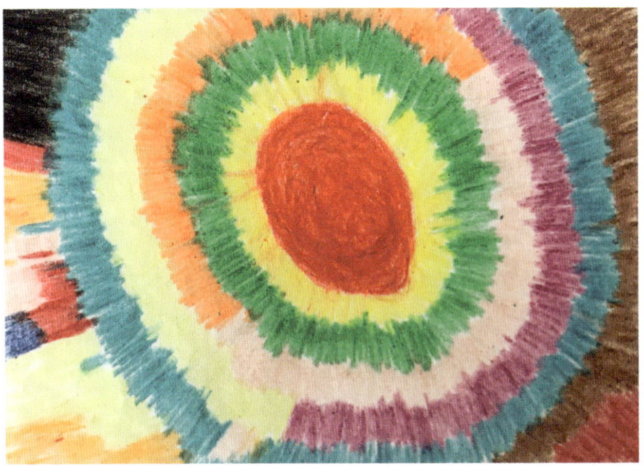

An explosion of colour and expression.

Alan went home for a while after his admission and spent some time with his family.

But sadly, his bone secondaries and pain got worse. He was admitted to the unit again, very unwell and in a lot of pain. An epidural catheter was put into Alan's back to control his pain. But he was deteriorating and clearly would die very soon. Although confused at times, he made it very clear that he wanted to be at home. This seemed impossible. An ambulance journey to his rural home along bumpy roads would be excruciating for him.

And then someone suggested the rescue helicopter service, a relatively new service to the region. Impossible. Transporting patients home is definitely not something they do. However someone in Alan's community pointed out that his father had been instrumental in the fund raising effort that bought the air ambulance. What's the harm in asking?

To everyone's surprise the answer was "yes". The proviso was, of course, that Alan's planned transfer home would have to be postponed if a community emergency occurred. Although this did happen once, the day came when Alan was eventually taken to the helipad on the roof of the hospital. He was safely tucked into the helicopter and flown home to the place he so loved.

Alan died 22 hours later.

The next day I went to visit Alan's home and he looked so peaceful. His bedroom had an amazing view over green hills of the family farm.

Not long after Alan's death I was asked to speak to a group of doctors and nurses about the use of impromptu drawings as a communication tool. As I sat and looked at the many pictures that people had drawn and given to me, I had another look at Alan's. The hairs on the back of my neck stood on end and my jaw dropped open. I hadn't noticed it before and it hadn't figured in the discussion that Alan and I had had about his picture. But there in the top righthand corner (which in Elisabeth's words tends to represent the near future) on top of the hospital was a *helicopter*!

It seemed that Alan's psyche had known.

The extent to which this young man had challenged and educated the whole team was huge, and so much that I now know I learnt from him on so many levels.

And so, thank you, Alan. Thank you for helping us to refine how we functioned as a team and how we could best serve you and others.

[1] Elisabeth Kübler-Ross would work with impromptu drawings with many thousands of grieving and dying people. A piece of A4 and a box of crayons was all that was required. She used this as a communication aid when words were difficult, or in fact, when there were no words at all. She could help people identify issues in their unconscious like no other.

One of the techniques that Elisabeth used with impromptu drawings was to ask the artist to draw on the paper using a landscape orientation. This would be the only instruction.

Her teachings revealed that by viewing the completed picture, it seemed that what was drawn (quite unconsciously) in each quadrant represented a different period of time. The images drawn in the lower left quadrant were about past events. The lower right quadrant represented future events. The upper right quadrant predicted the immediate future and the upper left quadrant the distant future, sometimes with information about the artist's death.

When working with people and impromptu drawings I generally haven't found this particular technique very helpful. However, Alan's picture did seem to have distinctly different images in each of the corners and Elisabeth's theory certainly seemed to work in this case.

Chapter 9

THAT WHICH CANNOT BE EXPLAINED

The more I have worked with people towards the end of life, the more I am in awe of the experiences people describe that seem to transcend intellectual explanation. It has made me acknowledge and examine my own spiritual beliefs and honour the vastness of that which we cannot explain.

My experiences with Maria and Simon illustrate some of the wonder of the inexplicable.

Spiritual connection

Maria

The first time I walked into her room I was struck by Maria's presence and mana. Maria was dying and had been in the inpatient palliative care unit for about a week.

I introduced myself and, as I sat down beside the bed, I looked up at the wall across the room. There was a large poster of a magnificent looking Native American chief. In the lower part of the poster were the words of the Native American Ten Commandments. I must have looked surprised because Maria immediately looked a little embarrassed.

'He's wonderful, isn't he?' I said.

'Yes,' Maria said shyly. 'I feel we Māori are very connected to North American Indians.' She then looked at me sideways and said, 'That chief often guides me.' She pointed at the poster and became really animated. 'Sometimes when I am just not sure what to do I look at the poster and it's almost as if the chief is guiding me, and telling me what decision I should make. I even asked him whether it would be the right thing to have my cancer chemotherapy. As soon as I looked at him, I knew I had to go ahead.' Maria then quickly remembered herself and said, 'Of course that's probably all nonsense and people will think I am mad.'

She thought that I would judge her for having such a belief and sense of spiritual connection.

I laughed and said, 'Well, you and me both. I have almost the same poster in my house and feel very connected to the Cherokee.'

Was it appropriate to share an experience of my own? I really don't know but it seemed very natural in that moment to share a connection I had often inexplicably felt with Cherokee.

I told her about an experience of driving in the United States. I was driving from Tennessee through North Carolina. At one part of the journey a strange feeling of fear, close to panic, came over me. I couldn't explain it and there was certainly no obvious reason for me to feel scared. Almost as suddenly as it came, it left. I shook it off and dismissed the memory of the feeling. However, driving back along the same route the panicky feeling returned for the same part of the road. Later I was reading a little more about the history of the region. It became clear that the piece of road on which I had experienced these feelings had been part of the Cherokee Trail of Tears. This is so-called because it was the route the Cherokee had been forced to take when driven from their lands. Many had died.

Maria looked at me and smiled knowingly.

With this sharing, it seemed that Maria and I connected at a deeper level. In the days that followed I was then able to support her in a more meaningful way. If she was mad then so was I.

This showed me how important it is to acknowledge the spiritual and belief systems of others without judgement.

Maria taught me to have courage to speak about such experiences while still maintaining a carefully respected boundary; one's sharing of beliefs needs to be helpful and supportive with no element of pushing one's own. A fine line this can be.

It certainly, for me, emphasises the importance of continual self-reflection and awareness as a clinical responsibility.

Nature

Simon

Jean and Simon were a close couple in their fifties with an understanding and connection that I really admired. They and their two children loved the outdoors and all had described a real love of nature.

Unfortunately, however, Simon had advanced cancer, and needed to be admitted to the palliative care inpatient unit where I was working in Sydney. When admitted his symptoms had been uncontrolled. He was more comfortable now but clearly very unwell and approaching the end of his life. Jean was there, sitting holding Simon's hand, when I visited one day.

'Has Simon told you about his owl?' she asked. I was intrigued.

'No, please do tell!' I said.

Simon looked at Jean with a shy smile.

'Well, as you know, I was pretty much housebound for the last three weeks before I came in here. Had to spend a lot of time in bed,' he said with a sigh. 'But one of the weird things is that an owl would come and sit on the tree just outside the window every evening. At first

I thought it was just a coincidence that he came three evenings in a row. But after a week I really came to feel he was coming to visit me. I really looked forward to his visit! The kids noticed too and even took his photo.'

Simon looked pensive. 'When I saw him sitting there it was as if he was trying to reassure me or something. Sounds a bit stupid but I always felt calmer when I saw him there.'

'It's quite odd,' Jean added. 'Simon has been in here a week now and the kids have looked for the owl each evening but they haven't seen him at all. It's as if he was just there for Simon.'

It was three days later that Simon died, a little unexpectedly. He had likely developed a pulmonary embolism, or blood clot in the lung, not uncommon in the final stages of advanced cancer. Fortunately, Jean was with him at the time.

About two weeks after Simon had died, I received a card from Jean acknowledging the support that the palliative care team had given to Simon, Jean and their two children. In the card was a photo of an owl. Jean explained that this was the photo they had taken when Simon had been at home. Apparently, the owl had not been seen while Simon was an inpatient but it had visited outside Simon's bedroom at home the evening that he died. His children had been home and seen it sitting in the tree in its usual place for just a few minutes before it flew away.

Seeing the owl had given them a sense of reassurance and peace.

'It was as if the owl had returned to let us know that somehow Simon was OK.'

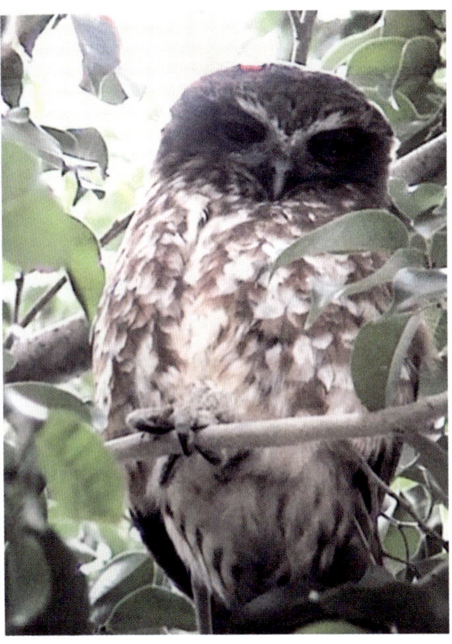

Simon's family were not traditionally religious. However they loved nature and spending time bush walking. Simon's connection to the owl, it seemed, had been a deeply spiritual experience.

Maria's and Simon's experiences reminded me again how important it is to acknowledge and validate all aspects of the human experience: the physical, emotional, intellectual, and the spiritual.

Chapter 10

COURAGE, DETERMINATION AND SERENITY

Elisabeth encouraged a focus on living until the moment of death rather than a focus on dying. Some people have the ability to do just this with courage, determination and serenity. The following are the stories of three such people.

Determination, humour and rebellion

Nancy

'John and I are going on a four-day cruise around New Zealand.'

'That will be lovely,' I said, humouring her.

Nancy was sitting in her garage on her hospital bed. She was gasping for breath and smoking a cigarette.

Nancy was a 55-year-old Maori woman whom I was visiting regularly with Carol, her community palliative care nurse. She had longstanding advanced lung disease and now also had lung cancer. The cancer had spread to her bones and liver and she had decided to have no more cancer treatment.

Her shortness of breath was helped by oxygen, of which she had a home supply. With oxygen, smoking is, of course, forbidden. And so, the bed was set up for her in the garage attached to the house. The garage was well lined, with a square of carpet on the floor so it was actually quite comfortable. With the garage roller door up Nancy had a view from her bed of paddocks and hills. The oxygen was kept inside the house. When she got really short of breath she would struggle into the house on her walker and gasp on the oxygen. No amount of discussion and cajoling would have Nancy give up her "ciggies".

'What's the point in giving them up now?' she would say. And who could argue with that? And reporting this to the service that supplied the oxygen didn't seem fair. The oxygen helped so much when she used it. Often this was at night and so she tended to sleep inside the house. So it worked out that Nancy was getting the symptom management she was prepared to accept, which in turn gave her some sense of being in control.

Nancy had an impish sense of humour and would often regale us with stories of her life before she became so sick. She had been into rally driving and one day greeted us dressed in her old rally driving jacket, covered in emblems. She modelled it proudly with her characteristic grin and sparkling eyes.

She would frequently come up with plans of what she would like to do and places she would like to visit, from going rally driving to flying to Australia for a holiday. And now she was telling us that she and her husband John were going on a cruise.

'It's going to be great!' she said excitedly. 'There will be a band and lots of dancing!'

'Sounds great,' I said. Carol and I left smiling knowingly at each other and shaking our heads.

However, the next time we visited Nancy, she told us that they were going next week and it was all arranged.

Her husband, John, was present and confirmed it. I think my mouth dropped open. Carol, sounding very shocked, said, 'But what about your oxygen?'

'Oh, they have oxygen on the ship! It's a big boat, you know!'

Once Carol and I had got over the initial shock of this announcement we talked to them about the wisdom of this trip. Had they thought about getting to the cruise ship and the need for portable oxygen for that journey? And what if Nancy suddenly got worse on the cruise? Some of the discussion was held with both Nancy and John together and some with John alone.

But Nancy was determined, John a little wary. They would have a letter with her laying out her medical history and requirements and would let the cruise ship know that she needed oxygen at times.

Carol and I were still sceptical that she would actually make the trip. If she did manage it, we couldn't imagine it being very enjoyable.

What did we know? When we saw Nancy nearly two weeks later, she was exhausted and clearly deteriorating. She was much shorter of breath and generally much frailer. However, she greeted us beaming. John nodded his head. John looked exhausted but was happy that he had managed to fulfil, in the last weeks of her life, his wife's long held desire to go on a sea cruise.

'I had the best time ever,' she said. 'I danced on the last night until one o'clock in the morning!'

Determination in spite of all odds

Joe

Joe was 41 years old and had come to live in Sydney from Vietnam some 10 years before.

He had only about half of one lung that functioned. He was in the inpatient palliative care unit to try and help his awful shortness of breath and pain.

'I'm ok,' he would say stoically whenever he was asked about his symptoms. My heart went out to this young man with this very rare type of lung cancer. 'I'll be fit enough to go and visit my mum in Vietnam soon,' he said brightly. He had just weeks to live. We had talked openly about this with him and his wife, Mai, but he just brushed it off.

He went home after about ten days, more comfortable, but still very short of breath. He managed his symptoms with medications and bloody mindedness. The community palliative care team were seeing him about twice a week for about three weeks. Then one day, they reported that they couldn't find him.

Someone suggested that he might be staying somewhere with friends. Maybe he had returned to Vietnam? We dismissed this as impossible, knowing how sick he was. We assumed that he would get in touch when he needed help.

About a week later I was going to Manila in the Philippines, where I was helping in the development of a palliative care programme. My flight would take me through Singapore. I was sitting at Sydney airport having a cup of coffee with my husband before the journey. The café was very close to Singapore Airlines' check-in. I thought my eyes were deceiving me. I saw Joe there. 'He must be seeing someone off,' I said to my husband.

But no, he was checking in. What should I do? I knew he was not fit to fly and, knowing his lung capacity, feared he might die on an international flight. Should I intervene? Should I alert the airline?

'Settle down,' I told myself. 'You have no right to do that. It would be a gross breach of his privacy.' With many feelings of disquiet, I finished my coffee, said goodbye to my husband and went through customs and security.

By the time I boarded the plane I had let go of the concern and told myself that Joe would have let the airline know what his needs were.

Ha! That's what I thought. I got up to go back to the toilet about an hour into the flight and saw Joe and Mai sitting about five rows behind me. As I moved down the aisle Mai greeted me enthusiastically.

'We're going back to Vietnam to see Joe's mother.'

'Yes,' said Joe, 'She has high blood pressure and can't fly!' I think my jaw fell open.

'Have you told the airline about your illness?' I asked them. The blank look told me that they had not.

'I think you better tell the flight attendants,' I said. 'You might need oxygen.'

'I'll be right,' said Joe. 'Don't want to make a fuss. I feel ok.' I imagined the fuss that would happen if Joe collapsed. But they were adamant and I didn't want to get into a discussion in front of other passengers.

'We've got all Joe's meds,' said Mai cheerfully. 'So, he'll be ok.'

When I got back to my seat I agonised over what I should do. I knew Joe could collapse and even die during the flight. However, after arguing with myself I again concluded that I didn't have the right to breach their confidentiality and interfere. I comforted myself with the knowledge that if something happened at least, as his palliative medicine specialist, I could respond and give advice.

It was a long flight.

When we arrived in Singapore I saw Joe there in a wheelchair. He looked terrible. He was planning to continue on to Vietnam and I to Manila. I was sure that this would be the last time I would see Joe. So, I gave him a hug and wished him well for the rest of his journey.

Two weeks later, I returned home and Joe's community palliative care nurse asked whether I could go and see Joe at home. He had made the journey back from Vietnam. I could not believe it.

His quiet determination made his journey possible. I admired this so much together with the serenity with which Joe was living. He was not focussing on dying. He was living until his heart stopped.

Determined to see her bucket list complete

Maryanne

I first met Maryanne and her old dog Sally in their caravan. They were in a rural camping ground in New Zealand where they had been staying for the last three weeks.

'I've come south to work on my "bucket list"', she announced with a smile. Maryanne had very advanced cancer with bone secondaries which were giving her pain. She had lost a lot of weight and was becoming quite frail. Maryanne had travelled from her home further north because she knew that her time was short. She had always been a bit of a loner, did not have a partner and had no children. But she had Sally, from whom she was inseparable.

Apparently, she had spent many happy years as a child and teenager in this quiet, beautiful part of the country. It had been her dream to return to the places she remembered and that was exactly what she was doing with her best friend before she died.

But Sally was sick too and Maryanne was determined not to die before her friend. After all, who would look after her? Maryanne quipped one day to a team member 'Perhaps we could jump off a cliff together!' It was said in jest, but had the team member very concerned when Maryanne appeared to be uncontactable for a few days.

However, Maryanne made contact from a tiny town, and the nurse went to see her there.

Both patients were deteriorating and eventually, Maryanne agreed to park her caravan not far from the hospice inpatient unit. She might need to be admitted quite soon. But again, Sally was her priority.

Eventually Maryanne's symptoms made it impossible for her to look after herself in the caravan. Yet she still refused to be admitted to the unit because of Sally. However, the hospice agreed that Sally could come too. The layout of the building made this possible with the large single rooms on the ground floor. The vet was arranged to visit Sally and so both received the care they needed and deserved.

Sadly, but also fortunately, Sally deteriorated and died before Maryanne. Maryanne's last days were filled with grief. But she did have the knowledge that she had honoured her commitment to her friend. Also, she had completed her "bucket list".

After Sally died, Maryanne and I talked more about the places that she and Sally had visited in the last weeks and how important this had been for her. 'It wasn't always easy,' she reflected. 'In fact at times it was bloody uncomfortable'. She sighed. 'But I am so pleased I did it!' And her eyes sparkled.

These three people have remained etched in my memory. They demonstrated so clearly the absolute power of courage and determination. Each lived fully despite a dire diagnosis and knowledge that their lives would be cut short.

Chapter 11

MESSING UP

Physician-assisted Suffering

It is often when situations didn't go well or when mistakes have occurred that we can learn the most. Sometimes we need to swallow our pride and honestly examine where we went wrong and could have done better. Self-awareness and reflection are imperative. I believe it is my personal responsibility as a healthcare professional to constantly examine my interactions and reactions. It is equally important for clinical teams to also honour this process.

The following are some stories where things did not go as well as they could. There were times when I wished

I had acted or responded differently. My unresolved issues had interfered with good rapport and empathy. There were also times when it seemed other team members' behaviour needed reflection.

She REALLY annoyed me

Linda

Linda was an attractive young woman in her late twenties, confined to bed and needing constant nursing care. She smiled brightly at me as I came into her room. Her mother, Judith, was sitting beside her.

'Hello Linda,' I said, 'My name's Sue. I've just joined the team.' I didn't get any further with my introduction when she burst into tears.

'Go away!' she said. Judith looked at me sadly.

'Ok,' I said, 'I'll come back a bit later.' I left the room wanting to also catch up with Linda's husband, Luke, who I knew was in the lounge.

I walked into the lounge where Luke was with Jamie, the couple's seven-year-old son. Luke appeared cheerful and very attentive to his young son. It was after school and on the way home Luke had brought Jamie in to see his mum. My heart went out to this young man who was juggling his job, looking after his son and making sure that they came to see Linda.

'I try to come as often as I can,' said Luke with a sigh. 'It's really hard. I actually feel a bit shut out by Linda's mum. Don't want to make waves though, cos we really couldn't have managed without her.'

They left quite soon after saying goodbye to Linda, with Jamie running and dancing out the door as only a seven-year-old does. I went back into Linda's room after Luke and Jamie left. Judith's look was thunderous and she let fly.

'That Luke is completely selfish! How dare he just bounce in and out like that! He's always out enjoying himself while Linda's just lying here!'

I took an immediate dislike to this woman. How dare she speak about that lovely young man like that. How did she think it was for him? Her vitriol did seem to dissipate quite quickly but our conversation remained stilted. I tried to include Linda.

'She can't answer your questions,' Judith snapped.

Linda had a brain tumour and was in the inpatient unit where I had just joined the team as clinical leader. Her cancer had been diagnosed six years previously when her young son was a few months old. A slow-growing tumour, it was initially removed successfully, but had recurred several times despite multiple surgical, radiotherapy and chemotherapy treatments. She was now in the palliative care inpatient unit. Her symptoms needed to be managed and her future care planned. Linda was completely unable to care for herself. She seemed alert but her ability to converse or take part in decisions was limited. She had become childlike; her emotions labile.

I learned that Linda and Luke had been teens together and married about eight years ago. Their happiness had seemed complete when Jamie was born a year later. But this was shattered when Jamie was just a few months old. As time went on, with each recurrence, Linda became more debilitated, and less and less able to take part in Jamie's care.

After my first meeting with Linda and Judith, our next interactions were more pleasant. I tried to remain empathetic and compassionate toward this mother who was losing her daughter.

However, Judith seemed to take every opportunity to criticise Luke. 'He should be here more! He's just out enjoying himself with Jamie! He's never been much of a husband!'

She didn't seem to be able to say anything good about this young man who had watched his bride gradually disappear before his eyes.

How dare she. I couldn't stand the woman. And so, I spent as little time as possible with her, choosing times to see Linda when Judith wasn't there. And just as bad, I started to find Linda's simpering, needy and childish demeanour irritating as well. Great.

My unconscious response was to spend less and less time with both Linda and Judith.

Consciously, I reasoned that there were others in the team who were better placed to support them. I advised on symptom management issues. But I kept my distance, more than I realised.

Once Linda's symptoms were stable, we needed to find a place for her continued care. Given her nursing needs, home was not an option. The team had conversations with Linda, Judith and Luke. Judith made it quite clear that she did not want her daughter moved. She found it hard to understand why Linda could not stay where she was.

The team spent a lot of time convincing Judith and Linda that the move would not be detrimental to Linda's care. Luke didn't seem to care. He had seemed to separate himself from Linda more and more during the time she was in the unit. I understood this as his way of grieving and the need to focus on their son.

Eventually the team social worker found an aged care facility that would care for Linda. And so, she was transferred.

Ten days later I had a call from Judith. She hated the care that Linda was now receiving. 'They don't seem to care and they don't have enough nurses,' cried Judith. 'She needs to come back. You must let her.'

'If you are concerned about Linda's care,' I said, 'you need to talk to the director of nursing there and the doctor looking after Linda.' I agreed to talk to our community palliative care team who visited the facility to give it support and advice.

A few days later, another call from Judith. I was annoyed that she had managed to get my number. She begged me to have Linda transferred back to the unit.

She said that Linda had a temperature and might have a urinary tract infection. This was very likely as Linda had an indwelling catheter and a urine infection is a common complication. I told Judith that if that was so it could easily be managed in the care facility and that the doctor looking after her would deal with it.

I brushed her off, saying, 'Linda is under his care now. If he thinks her symptoms are unstable enough then he can always refer her back here for readmission.'

A week later came the news that Linda had developed septicaemia and died.

And the guilt hit me. Finally, but too late, I reflected on what had been happening from the moment I had met Judith.

Certainly, the healthcare system had let Linda and her family down in that there was a lack of facilities that specifically took care of young people with long term needs.

Had our team failed to provide the ongoing support that the team had promised when Linda was transferred?

However most shocking for me was the recognition that when I had first met Judith, I had been really annoyed by her. This was a woman who was grieving about what was happening to her beloved daughter. Your child is not supposed to die before you. It is the wrong order of things. Why had I let her behaviour get to me?

Something about her had awakened in me a past experience. This had then interfered with my ability to give the empathy and compassion she deserved. Thus, I contributed to her suffering.

What was this about? It was to do with her venom and unfairness towards Luke. And then I remembered.

Some years earlier a friend had asked me to help with the palliative care of his 25-year-old daughter, Jane. She was returning home to New Zealand from Australia as she was dying. I helped with her transfer from Australia and admitted her briefly to the hospital inpatient unit where I worked. She was then going to her mother's home in another town. Jane's parents had apparently had a very acrimonious divorce years earlier and still barely spoke.

I never did work out why, but the day that Jane was about to be discharged from the unit her mother barged into my office.

'How dare you!' she said. 'Your behaviour has been completely unethical.'

'What do you mean?' I asked.

'You know! You should be ashamed! Conniving with him!' I guessed she was referring to Jane's father but I had no idea what she was talking about.

'If you have a complaint perhaps you need to talk with the manager,' I said, really puzzled.

'Don't you tell me what to do!' she said, as she flounced out of the office.

I felt shocked and traumatised as I really had no idea at the time what it was about. It felt so unfair. Judith's unfairness towards Luke and the aggression with which she spoke awakened in me the indignation about the unfair judgement I had experienced from Jane's mother.

And so, an unresolved issue or "unfinished business" had been evoked, interfering with the support I was able to give Judith at one of the worst times in her life. My consequent lack of compassion almost certainly added to her distress and suffering.

How different this might have been if I had reflected on my initial reaction to Judith sooner …

Please help me!

Leno

Leno's wide eyes looked at me pleadingly. He was sitting on a dilapidated chair at the doorway of the room he shared with five other men. The room had three beds. His chest was heaving trying to get air into his lungs.

Leno was 30 years old and dying of pulmonary tuberculosis in the Infectious Diseases Hospital for the poor in Manila. He came from the provinces and like many of the patients in the crowded ward, he had been abandoned here. Relentless poverty meant that families could not afford to care for those who were non-productive. Medications were expensive and, even if provided free, the extra care needed was beyond their means. There was also the social stigma and fear of the diagnosis of tuberculosis.

Even worse, Leno had MDR (multi-drug resistant) tuberculosis. If he was to have any chance of treatment, he needed special drugs not available at this hospital.

He looked up at me, 'Please, ma'am!' How I hated that title which to me reeked of class distinction. 'PLEASE! Will you help me?'

Leno's huge desperate eyes still haunt me.

'I'm sure that the doctors here are doing all that they can for you,' I said lamely. I felt completely helpless. The drugs that might help him were available elsewhere at a price. He was asking me to advocate for him and try and procure the drugs for him. But I rationalised that I was a visitor to this hospital and this country and couldn't do anything, could I? And so, I left the ward.

I hadn't even sat with him to hear his anguish. I further rationalised that I shouldn't linger because of the risk of transmission.

After leaving the ward I felt really uncomfortable. Why was this? It was just very sad that this man was so sick and dying, I told myself. Anyone would feel uncomfortable.

I was visiting the hospital with two colleagues two to three times a year to help develop a palliative care programme at the hospital. The pulmonary tuberculosis ward was one of the saddest and most crowded wards.

Leno's face haunted me for days. This was about more than the normal reaction to a sad situation. Gradually I realised that my reluctance to get involved reflected a childhood fear. As a child if I made a fuss I risked getting into trouble as a result. There was also an old feeling of helplessness that I couldn't change the status quo.

Could I have tried to make a fuss and advocate for Leno? It may not have made any difference. But I will never know.

Once again, my old issues and learnt defence mechanisms had got in the way. My old fears had prevented me from being focussed on Leno and his distress.

And he was one of so many. The number of similar stories was overwhelming. It felt that there were just too many for my efforts to make any difference.

Then I remembered the Starfish story.

Soon after we first came to Manila to help in the development of a hospital palliative care team, there was a welcome ceremony. One of the dignitaries told us this story:

One day there had been a fierce storm by the sea. The beach was strewn with hundreds of starfish washed up, stranded and dying. An elderly monk was walking along and as he walked, he picked up a starfish and returned it to the sea. As he continued walking, he passed a young man going the other way.

'What you doing, old man?' said the young man, as the

monk bent down and picked up a starfish.

'I'm returning this starfish to the water so that it can live,' replied the monk.

The young man scoffed. 'You'll never make a difference. Just look how many there are!'

The young man walked on, shaking his head.

The monk bent down and picked up another starfish, and as he returned it to the sea he quietly said, 'Made a difference to that one!' [1]

At the time I had looked down and realised that the dress I was wearing was patterned all over with starfish.

After hearing this story, the fledgling palliative care team decided to call themselves the Starfish Palliative Care Team. This reminded them of the importance, despite apparent overwhelming numbers, of making a difference to just one person.

As I recalled the story, I felt ashamed of my response to Leno.

[1] Adapted from *The Star Thrower* by Loren Eiseley (1907–1977).

Secrecy, suspicion and collusion

Renata

It was my first visit to Renata, 36 years old and a mother for the first time. She lived in a small cramped apartment with her husband, Marko, and their two-month-old son Joseph.

'I keep losing my balance,' she said. I was immediately alarmed. Had she got brain secondaries?

I knew that Renata had liver and bone secondaries from breast cancer but this new symptom was particularly worrying. She had developed a large breast lump about three years ago. It was an aggressive cancer but initially there was no obvious spread. However, Renata, a structural engineer, wanted more information and opinions. She wanted to know as much as she could before embarking on treatment. She was also very suspicious of the motives of her advisors. She thus initially refused what was recommended and sought multiple opinions. It was a year later before she agreed to treatment. By then the cancer was larger and had spread to the lymph nodes.

'I'm scared I might drop Joseph,' she confided. I shared her concern.

'Tell me about what's been happening,' I said. 'I know you had your original breast cancer treated a bit more than two years ago …' Before I could continue, she interrupted.

'You mustn't tell Marko that!' She looked scared. What did she mean?

Apparently, she had met Marko about six months after her cancer treatment had finished and hadn't told him about her cancer. They married shortly afterwards and within a short time she became pregnant.

'The oncologist said it would be alright to get pregnant,' she exclaimed. I doubted this very much but that was what she believed.

Towards the end of her pregnancy, Renata had developed severe back pain which heralded the diagnosis of widespread cancer by the time her baby was just two months old.

She commenced hormone treatment to try and slow down the disease. The oncologist then referred her to the community palliative care service for symptom management and support.

The situation was dire; a mother with very advanced cancer and a husband who was completely overwhelmed.

Why had his wife developed such widespread cancer so suddenly? Renata swore the team to secrecy concerning her diagnosis before she had met Marko. Neither Renata nor Marko had any other family to support them. They had each come to Australia alone from Eastern Europe to try and seek better lives. They had both left a homeland that had seen the terrible ravages of conflict with families divided against each other. Suspicion kept you alive.

The palliative care inpatient unit admitted Renata with Joseph, to try and improve her symptoms and support the young family.

My suspicions were unfortunately correct. Renata had developed multiple brain secondaries and the treatment options were very limited. She had increasing visual problems and headaches due to the swelling around the many secondaries in her brain. Steroid medication was commenced to reduce swelling around the brain secondaries and help the symptoms they were causing. Radiotherapy was recommended to give the best chance of slowing the growths. Two radiation oncologists gave this same opinion. Having practised as a radiation oncologist before moving to palliative medicine, I added my support to this opinion.

Renata was having none of it.

Despite all the oncology opinions that surgery was just not possible, Renata was adamant that she wanted a neurosurgical opinion. That, we agreed to arrange.

'But you are not to give the neurosurgeon any information about me,' she said.

'But …,' I started to say.

'No! I want his opinion to be completely independent. I don't want him to know what you all think!'

Marko was completely overwhelmed by all of this and looked lost. I was frustrated. Delaying treatment would be disastrous. We knew that the neurosurgeon would not contemplate surgery. And, of course, no surgeon would see a patient without *any* information being provided.

Eventually we persuaded Renata that surgery was not possible and that radiotherapy had the best chance of improving her symptoms. Radiotherapy could help her headaches and stop her sight from worsening so that she could spend some comfortable weeks with her baby and husband.

At the same time, Renata had a follow-up appointment with her medical oncologist. He had previously told the palliative care team caring for her that further chemotherapy would be futile and, in fact, would likely cause awful side effects. However, she was demanding it and he decided to treat her. My frustration felt boundless.

Chemotherapy would delay radiotherapy to her brain secondaries. Chemotherapy and nowadays immunotherapy are vital treatments in the management of cancer. But in these circumstances? It seemed that Renata's medical oncologist just could not face telling her the truth. Renata had very extensive disease and her ability to tolerate aggressive chemotherapy was dubious. This medical oncologist promoted himself as an expert and taught communication skills. And yet, he seemed unable to be truthful with Renata and colluded with the notion that chemotherapy might help her.

Meanwhile, Renata and her baby remained in the inpatient palliative care unit. There were some concerns as to whether she was able to care for the baby safely. When they were first admitted, the nurses were happy to support Renata in caring for her baby, especially as Marko was often there, having given up his construction job.

However, the charge nurse returned from leave and was adamant that having the baby in the unit was not safe and was not within their "nursing scope of practice". She was known to be somewhat inflexible and, along with other staff, my frustration flared. How could she call herself a caring palliative care nurse? There was no point in attempting to discuss the issue with her. Certainly, she and I had not seen eye to eye on a number of occasions.

Joseph went home with his father.

A few days later Renata was transferred to the care of her medical oncologist and received chemotherapy. She deteriorated quickly and died when Joseph was little more than four months old.

Many members of the team were left feeling that they hadn't been able to serve Renata, Marko and Joseph as well as they would have liked. I know that was so for me. Had I let my lack of understanding Renata's background get in the way? My frustration and even indignation with both her and Marko were very real at times. What was that about in me? Why had I not reflected on those more at the time. Perhaps I could have become clearer about my issues that were being awakened so that, in turn, I could then be more present for them.

Renata had been brought up in a country which had

been torn apart by conflict and to survive one needed to be wary and suspicious. Her suspicion of the medical profession and opinions that were given to her was so understandable. How could she trust that they didn't have agendas other than her wellbeing? Had those caring for her understood this enough? Had I?

And then there were clearly the wider team issues. What was making the charge nurse so inflexible? How could that have been better addressed? Perhaps it couldn't.

The collusion of the oncologist and his inability to be truthful in giving bad news was obvious. Was his reluctance to be honest really about Renata's needs? Or did it reflect his own unresolved issues around death and perhaps even a need to be heroic?

And once again, had my old defence mechanism of "don't make a fuss" kicked in? Could I have been more assertive with the medical oncologist?

So many questions and causes for reflection …

How we interact with the people we seek to serve tells us much about ourselves, our strengths and our weaknesses. Understanding why we react in certain ways, becoming more aware of our defence mechanisms, will allow us to respond more openly and honestly. Otherwise, there is a danger of inflicting, what I have come to call, Physician-assisted Suffering. A constant commitment to self-reflection and self-awareness is a clinical responsibility.

Chapter 12

SELF-CARE AS A CLINICAL RESPONSIBILITY

The Wounded Healer

'Put your own oxygen mask on first before you try to help others.' The familiar aircraft safety briefing provides a good metaphor for self-care.

As I grew up, caring for yourself before looking after others would have been regarded as hedonistic and selfish. Always put other peoples' needs first was the dogma of the day. But there is now a large range of literature advocating self-care first.

Self-help books encourage balance in one's life; the need to balance work, a career, family, whānau, friends, community involvement, leisure, hobbies and, of course, maintaining one's own physical health are essentials of self-care.

Self-care. I interpret this as nurturing oneself physically, emotionally, intellectually and spiritually with a wider social component in all areas. However, often overlooked in self-care, particularly in a clinical setting, is the critical importance of self-awareness.

This is at the core of what I started to become aware of, and I was first introduced to it by Elisabeth Kübler-Ross and her team. 'If you want to work with the dying, deal with your own shit first.' When I first heard her say that, I did not have a clue what she meant. But … it started my journey of self-awareness.

We all have our "shit"; we all have our wounds.

The term "wounded healer" was coined by Henri Nouwen, psychologist in 1972, with the idea that the analyst treats patients because the analyst themself is "wounded". The origins can be traced to the centaur, Chiron, in Greek mythology who was indeed a "wounded healer". Carl Jung also encompassed the concept in his writings. Effective "wounded healers" need to acknowledge, explore and try to understand their woundedness. The term itself has been somewhat overused but, over time, I have come to appreciate the concept and tried to integrate its depth of meaning.

Elisabeth developed and described her holistic quadrant personality model. This is a useful way of examining how wounding and potential suffering can occur and accumulate as one develops.

Elisabeth had a gift for presenting information. She seemed to be able to distil the essence of others' teachings and communicate concepts like no one else I had ever heard.

One such piece of teaching is her Four Quadrant Personality Model. It incorporates the old wisdom of indigenous cultures and modern developmental theories and is elegant in its simplicity.

Very simply, this discusses the human personality as having four aspects: physical, emotional, intellectual and spiritual. These aspects develop from birth; they can flourish with good nurturing, but equally stunting and distortion can occur with neglect and abuse. Our woundedness accumulates over time.

Clearly it is but a model, not a rigid formula. As Jacob Watson wrote, it can be regarded as a diagnostic tool to clarify whether these four aspects are in balance. Over the years I have found it incredibly useful in helping me to try and achieve equilibrium in my life.

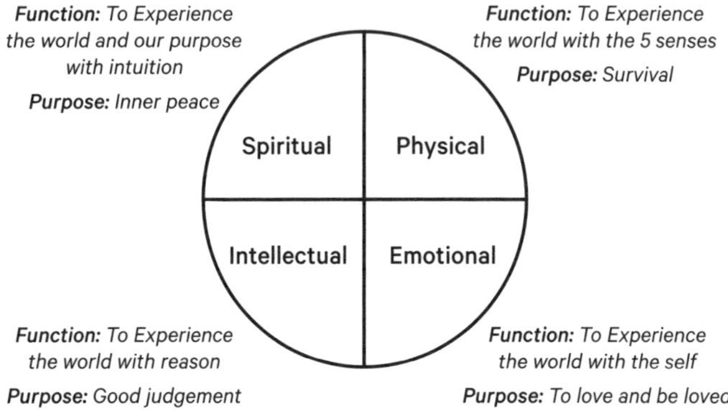

The physical quadrant is that part of us that experiences the world with our five senses and is responsible for survival.

The emotional quadrant is the personality aspect that experiences the world through connection and relationship with "Self". There is a need to belong, to love and be loved.

The intellectual quadrant experiences the world with reason and its purpose is to provide good judgement.

The part designated the spiritual quadrant can be regarded as that which experiences the world and our purpose with intuition. Its purpose is to achieve inner peace. This is the part of us, however, which is so personal that everyone will have their own way of explaining it.

The quadrants all interact, of course. Each affects the other. But it can be useful to look at the aspects separately as an aid to understanding the role of each.

In this model, all quadrants are present at birth and maybe even from conception, depending on your belief system. However, there does seem to be an emphasis on maturation in each quadrant at certain ages.

This photo was taken shortly after my first granddaughter was born.

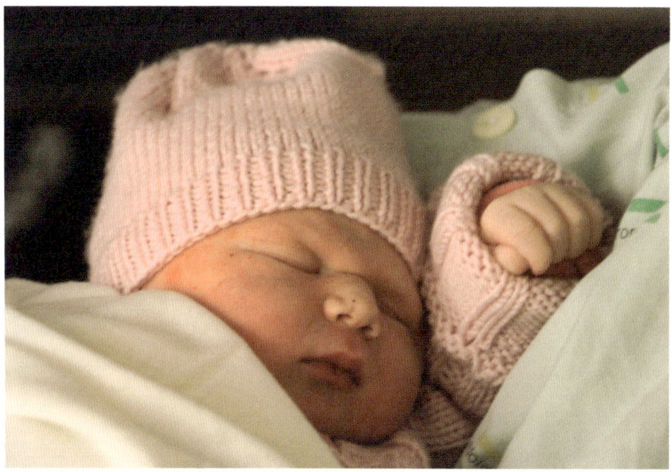

For me, it is an image of the innocence and potential of a newly born human. The challenge is to nurture this new human being in all aspects.

So, how do these aspects develop and flourish? And how, unfortunately, does suffering develop and create our woundedness?

From birth, the needs of the physical quadrant are immediate, vital and evident with an accompanying big increase in physical growth. From birth, a little one needs touch and to be kept dry, clean, warm and fed as primary needs. Ask any parent how quickly a little one grows out of clothes in the first three months. The first three months sees a doubling of size. That is not to say, of course, that there is not emotional, intellectual and spiritual presence and growth at this time, but the immediate and initial imperative is good physical nurturing.

Sadly, however, many little ones in our world do not get this critical physical nurturing. They may not get the food they need, the shelter or the touch that they require. They do not thrive. In our world, also, not only are our little ones physically neglected but they may be physically and sexually abused.

I often feel haunted by the pictures of children we

see from impoverished and conflict zones in the world. Stunting of growth is obvious and there is fear and sadness in their faces.

And we see this close to home. Cathy's story comes to mind. The neglect and the physical and sexual abuse that she suffered growing up stayed as body memory throughout her life and affected her responses.

Many of us may experience less obvious neglect and physical insult as we grow. But they can still cause and create unconscious responses in later life.

One of my physical responses to stress and anxiety was to start coughing. During the course of my own inner journeying, I discovered that it was my body memory of a horrific early childhood experience. Becoming aware of, and working through, that event reduced my anxiety and that physical response.

Every parent is keen to experience that first smile from their little one. To me the first smiles represent an early conscious attempt at a relationship. The emotional quadrant is expanding. Ideally those smiles are mirrored back. Then, further smiles and interactions are exchanged.

With growth, that experience of being noticed and affirmed enhances trust and confidence that says 'Hey, I'm ok!' That child will feel accepted for who they are.

When we are sad, we need to cry. When we are angry, we need to be able to say 'No!' and may need to yell or even have a tantrum. When we are scared, we need to express that. When we are happy, we laugh and smile. If our emotions are allowed to be expressed, we are more likely to grow up acknowledging our true feelings. How we feel matters. When our natural emotions are not allowed their expression, they become repressed and over time distorted into more dangerous and destructive forces. Examples of this are rage and violence, anxiety, panic, phobias, self-condemnation, self-pity, some types of depression and many other emotions. Elisabeth described these distorted emotions as being like the making of a huge pool of unresolved feelings and issues. She called this "unfinished business".

Acceptance of who we are needs to be unconditional and not dependent on what we do. Such is unconditional love. But this needs to be accompanied by clear and consistent boundaries for behaviour. For example, it is normal to feel angry but it is not acceptable to hurt someone else or ourselves with our anger. Similarly, if there is a skill that we need to learn (for example tying our shoelaces) it can't be always done for us. We need to be encouraged to try.

Much wounding can occur as we grow when we are not accepted for who we are. We get the message that we must change to be accepted; that we have to "prostitute" ourselves to be loved. How often do we hear the emotional message, 'I love you if…' rather than simply 'I love you'. The adults in our life can be judgmental, dismissive and scornful and we can develop feelings of rejection, betrayal, abandonment and a poor sense of self-worth.

The significant adults in our life are, almost always of course, trying to do their best. It is very rare that they are trying to hurt or damage. But, their subconscious, unresolved issues, their "unfinished business", will get in the way and dictate behaviour.

Trauma in early life can result in us developing defences to try and keep us safe. We may bury feelings and cover them with all sorts of defence mechanisms. These become subconscious and are designed to try and keep us from being hurt further. Early in my training with the Elisabeth Kübler-Ross team, one of the trainers pointed out to me that when I was in a stressful situation and seemed vulnerable, I appeared to dissociate.

'It is as if you disappear somewhere,' I was told. Initially I was puzzled as to what on earth they were talking about. With time, more internal journeying and psychotherapeutic help, I came to realise what this was about. Eventually I faced the trauma of some sexual abuse at a preverbal age. I realised that at that time, to survive the experience, I had dissociated. This formed my defence mechanism of "disappearing" whenever I felt in anyway threatened, especially in the presence of male authority. I had perfected this so well that I didn't know I was doing it.

If the physical and emotional quadrants are well nurtured the intellectual quadrant is very well set to flourish in its development. Hence children become avid for information and therefore become more prepared to take on further formal schooling. They need to be encouraged both in their sense of wonder to search for new knowledge and in their efforts to attempt new skills and tasks.

This can enhance a sense of possibility and confidence in attempting innovation.

Unfortunately, constant criticism and being told to do better can dampen self-worth. There may be over emphasis, for example, on rankings in school. This can lead to over-competitiveness and a need to win at all costs. Or, the opposite can result with feelings of being stupid or dumb. A sense of inadequacy or inferiority can result with a loss of heart and the wanting to give up. Why try? Suffering.

As children move into adolescence, expression of the spiritual quadrant becomes more evident. They start to ask the "big" questions. There is a curiosity of life's major dilemmas. Who or what is in charge? Why do bad things happen to people? Why do people have to suffer? What is important? They start questioning beliefs, customs and rituals. Support and encouragement when considering and struggling with these uncertainties is important. Reassurance and such support will nurture spiritual development.

In our society this does not always happen and young people can be left with a sense of pointlessness, despair and hopelessness. The sad statistics around suicide in young people are testament to this.

In Western societies there tends to be an emphasis on the physical and intellectual aspects of the personality. How one looks and what one does; how many qualifications one has is of the utmost importance. This is often at the expense of understanding and nurturing the emotional and spiritual aspects of oneself.

The quadrants can then look like this:

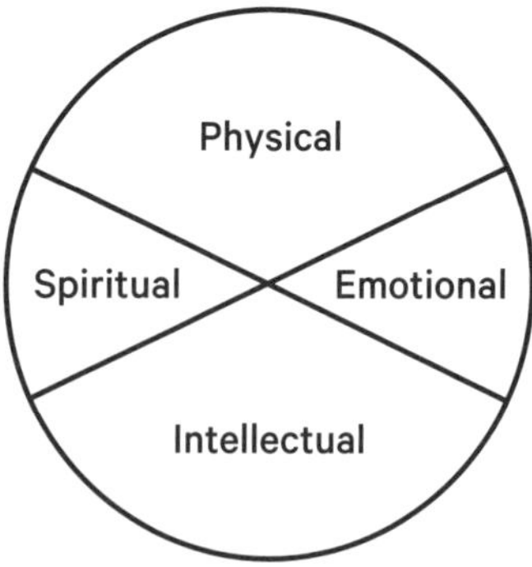

The goal of good nurturing in all quadrants is to achieve balance. Each quadrant needs regular attention and nurturing. When this happens, there is more opportunity to access and develop creativity and balanced growth.

A colleague always drew a spiral at the centre of the balanced quadrants. The spiral is a fundamental symbol in many cultures. It almost always symbolises growth or new beginnings. When the quadrants are in balance, creativity and growth are made more possible.

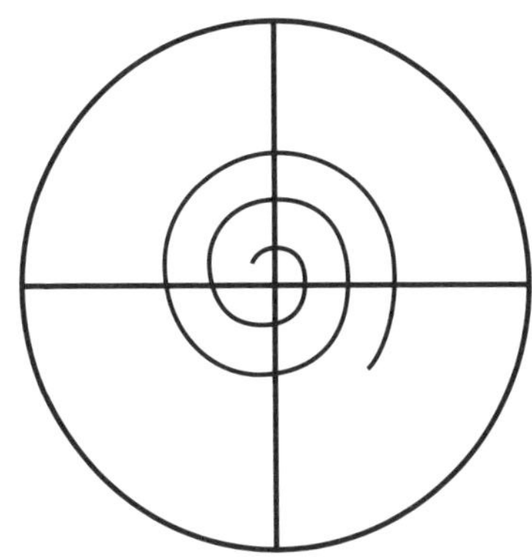

Mason Durie articulated the Māori perspective of "balanced whole person care" in his model Te Whare Tapa Whā.

Something is not right

Life, of course, is not ideal and at times we feel out of balance, stressed and overwhelmed.

It can be useful to use the quadrants to help recognise the signals in each quadrant before one begins to be overwhelmed. This can be a useful step in self-awareness. Viewed another way, we can recognise the symptoms or indicators that all is not well. Such indicators will be personal but here are some examples.

In the physical quadrant one may, for example, develop stiff shoulders, back aches, headaches, constant colds. The onset of insomnia may occur. Or the opposite may be an indicator that all is not well, i.e. sleeping too much. One may start overeating or stop eating. Libido may suddenly be lost. Over-drinking or indulgence in recreational drugs might occur. All of these can be viewed as indicators in the physical quadrant that all is not well, that we are in danger of being overwhelmed and not coping.

In the emotional quadrant one may become aware of being more irritable, judgmental, critical or sarcastic. One might notice becoming anxious, weepy or unsettled. Or the opposite may be true. There is a numbness. A loss of confidence may occur. Or one becomes aware of putting on a mask, e.g. smiling on the outside while crying inside. One might put on a tough or robotic front or a comedian's mask. Each person will have their own indicators of emotional "symptoms" that are personal and say, 'all is not well.'

An indicator in the intellectual quadrant can be that one starts becoming dogmatic; always right and not listening to others' opinions. Another might be the tendency to over rationalise and overthink situations. One may stop studying. Or the opposite may be true: studying without a break. Watching too much television may be an indicator. It may be that one gives up leisure reading or in fact the opposite: reading too many "trashy" novels.

In the spiritual quadrant one may become aware of a sense that life has lost meaning. There may be a sense of emptiness. One may notice a loss in the joy of nature. Spiritual or religious practices may become neglected, or practised excessively. A loss in the joy of music may be an indicator for some.

Each person will have their own indicators that are personal. Using this model can be a useful and simple guide to help bring awareness to oneself when something needs to change to achieve life balance. And of course, self-awareness requires one to be completely honest with oneself.

That is sometimes difficult. I have found it helpful to have people that I trust who are willing to point out, in a non-judgemental way, when there are changes in my behaviour. While I was trying to make sense of the feedback I had received about disappearing or dissociating, I found it really useful that my mentors could tell me when they observed it happening.

Nurturing and healing

The earlier that one becomes aware that all is not well, the better. With practice one can then avoid becoming overwhelmed. This is the first step to good nurturing and healing. Diagnosis needs to precede treatment.

Again, I have found it useful to use the four quadrant model and consider nurturing in each part.

In many ways the physical quadrant is the easiest to contemplate nurturing. One might consider needing more rest and/or sleep? Do I need to exercise more, e.g. walking, running, cycling, going to the gym? Would Yoga or Thai Chi help? Should I have a haircut, a facial or a massage? Do I need a medical check-up?

Each has their own way of nurturing the physical quadrant.

The emotional quadrant can be the toughest to examine honestly and to be able to decide on what is needed; to honour that, healing needs to take place. Taking time out to be still and to reflect may be the first step. The use of journaling one's innermost thoughts and feelings can be helpful. Some find taking notice of one's dreams useful and so too the use of "impromptu drawings". Artwork of any sort or one's hobbies can be very nurturing for the emotional self.

Perhaps the most important way of nurturing and healing the emotional quadrant is by seeking support.

Support may be from friends and family, work colleagues or from independent professionals.

The best support comes from those that we trust to hear what we are saying without judgement and without giving unsolicited advice. Sometimes we just need to offload and be heard. Other times we may ask for comment.

The support of friends, family and colleagues can be invaluable. However, to really work through emotional distress and difficulties it is useful to have professional help. To this end, healthcare professionals working in the area of emotional support very often have regular clinical supervision. This has been well known in the fields of psychology, psychotherapy, counselling and social work and in more recent years in palliative care. Clinical supervision in this sense is not the supervision of professional skills. Rather it is the opportunity for independent help and guidance in reflecting and healing the emotional impact of working with others in their suffering and distress.

One needs to have the courage and commitment to examine and become aware of one's own patterns of behaviour and understand what triggers one's personal and unique emotional responses. Then "burnout" and "compassion fatigue" are less likely to occur. And perhaps, even more important, one's own issues are less likely to get in the way of providing care and service.

The care that I wanted to provide to Anna (Chapter 2) was nearly compromised because I wasn't fully conscious of the loneliness in my own life. Fortunately, I recognised in time that something was being evoked in me that needed attention. Once I had worked through that with my supervisor, I was then better able to support Anna with her journey.

Not so with Linda's mother, Judith. I remained self-righteously angry, failed to listen to the warning within myself and rather than relieving suffering, I likely added to it.

Self-awareness in the emotional quadrant then involves becoming aware of our patterns of behaviour and understanding what triggers us. This then provides us with *protection* from burnout or compassion fatigue and reduces *projection* onto the situation before us.

The intellectual quadrant equally needs nurturing and may well be the part of us that gets overworked. Some suggested ways of nurturing this quadrant are relaxing with a good book or TV. Or it may be that more studying or journal reading is needed if this has been neglected. It may be that less is required. Some find crosswords or Sudoku helpful. Healthy debate or engaging in non-dogmatic discussion can be intellectually nurturing.

Again, this will be completely individual and depends on honesty with oneself.

Nurturing the spiritual quadrant will be as diverse as there are people on the earth. Some suggestions that people have found nurturing in this respect are taking a walk in nature, gardening, watching a sunset or sunrise, listening to music or singing. Meditating or resuming religious practice may be nurturing if this has been neglected.

And, of course, many activities or practices will provide nurturing in all four quadrants at the same time. All aspects are interconnected and are never separate in reality. But it can be helpful to consider and consciously focus on each part regularly.

When all four quadrants are equally considered, examined and nurtured, better balance is possible. This allows us to focus more completely on others' needs. Such focus and presence then allow healing and transcendence for those we seek to serve. Self-awareness becomes our clinical responsibility.

Some Personal Experiences of Attempting Self-awareness

Thank you, Elisabeth, again for introducing me to the importance of self-awareness or "dealing with my own shit first"!

Externalisation

Over the years I have continued to use the teachings and techniques learnt from Elisabeth and her team as well as other mentors and teachers.

Elisabeth's workshops were based on creating a safe place where there was no judgement. Absolute confidentiality was paramount. In such an environment one could be totally heard, perhaps for the first time. These workshops were originally developed by Elisabeth for the dying, to deal with their "unfinished business" as she called it. She recognised that the dying needed to be heard. Working through some of the emotional weight they were carrying allowed more peace at death. She quickly recognised that this was also true for everyone to actually live well. Dealing with unfinished business or unresolved issues of loss and grief allows us to live more fully and more peacefully. Her workshops were then opened to everyone. One of the most powerful aspects of these workshops was having healthcare professionals in the same room as those with life-threatening illnesses. Therein came the recognition of the universality of human suffering.

Elisabeth and her team used an externalisation process in the workshops but it was the creation of a completely safe and non-judgemental environment that I believe was the essence of the healing that occurred there. A sacred space was created and allowed the interplay of emotional and spiritual healing.

For the first time, at that first workshop, I gained a sense of why if something went wrong it always felt like my fault. I lived with a constant underlying feeling of guilt. If something didn't go quite right with a patient's treatment and they did not respond as had been hoped, it must be my fault. What I became aware of was that somehow I had a deep-seated sense that my father's illness had been my fault. Not logical but emotionally very real. My father had multiple sclerosis and was a very frustrated and angry man. Understandable perhaps, but the perception of a young girl growing up and often being the butt of his anger was that his disease and situation was her fault. Understanding this explained why if someone slipped on a banana skin, nowhere even near her, it was her fault. The insight gained made a huge difference from then on.

Hence, I embraced and learnt more of Elisabeth's concepts and teachings over a number of years and have always been grateful to her for friendships made and colleagues worked with while training with her organisation.

Impromptu Drawings

Through Elisabeth's workshop I also learnt the value of impromptu drawings both as another externalisation process and also as a tool when working with a therapist to delve deeper into the psyche. I was fortunate to meet Gregg Furth, a New York-based Jungian therapist, and take part in many of his workshops, furthering my understanding of impromptu drawings. I used the tool in my own self-awareness journey as well as working with people at the end of life. I am no technical artist but just using a box of crayons and pieces of A4 I would put my feelings onto paper. Doing a series of drawings over time would also give me a sense of my progress. Just recently, I had the sense of being overwhelmed and very vulnerable; that I was in a deep emotional well. After working with my supervisor, I decided to draw an impression of this, to include what might help me when the feeling became intense. The picture was no masterpiece but over the next few days I took it out and looked at it. Somehow it gave me the courage to know that healing was happening.

Clinical Supervision

Regular and skilled clinical supervision have proved to be an indispensable part of honouring my commitment to self-awareness as a clinical responsibility. In order to be effective, it has been important to make sure that the clinical supervisor I chose was right for me. I needed someone with whom I felt safe to be vulnerable in front of. But also, someone who would challenge my belief systems and prejudices. Over the years, depending on where I was working and my personal circumstances at the time, I have used psychotherapists, psychologists, psychiatrists, counsellors and a Jungian analyst as clinical supervisors. I am grateful to them all for their honesty and help.

At times the issues that I needed to work with were

emotional responses to clinical situations such as Anna's. Other times the issues were related to the healthcare settings in which I was working. When the hospital palliative care unit was closed, I felt betrayed. I felt helpless that I couldn't change what was happening. My supervisor helped me to untangle why I was feeling so traumatised. It was evoking a deep-seated old feeling. As a child I had not been able to change the bullying from my father. It was as if the hospital had taken on his persona. The second example occurred when I was working in a community setting. I was deeply concerned at processes and clinical practices that had developed. In my view, these jeopardised good patient care. My attempts to change this just resulted in acrimony, without change. This triggered feelings of indignation and helplessness. Working with my supervisor I decided that my integrity was being compromised. Making my concerns known, I resigned in both cases.

Talking Circles

The indigenous peoples of the world have such wisdom. In many cultures the power and value of a "talking circle" is well known. It relies on silently and attentively listening.

Forming a talking circle group can be supportive and nurturing. The friends or colleagues in the circle need to be those trusted to be non-judgemental and to respect absolute confidentiality. I have been lucky to be part of such a group. Traditional cultures often use a talking stick. The person who holds the stick has the authority to speak and no one interrupts or comments. Only when the speaker has finished is the stick passed on. In the circles to which I have belonged, we have used a stone but with the same idea. No comments or advice are given unless invited. Confidentiality is an absolute ground rule.

So often in our everyday life we are not given the space to speak from our heart and soul in a safe way. We are interrupted and we are given advice or told how we should feel. And our confidentiality is not respected. The adherence to and the mutual respect for the "unwritten contract" within the talking circle provides the sacred space that may be missing in our lives. It allows for us to be really heard.

Acupoint Tapping

Another modality that I have found increasingly helpful in my pursuit of self-care and self-awareness and working with distress and suffering has been the use of acupoint tapping.

I was first introduced to tapping using EFT (Emotional Freedom Technique) about 20 years ago by a psychotherapy colleague. Based on traditional Chinese medicine and developed by Gary Craig, EFT involves tapping on various acupressure points in the upper body while focussing on a particular emotional issue. There is usually a set up phrase based on the issue stated at the beginning and the tapping is done in a certain order.

To someone trained in traditional Western medicine with a radiation oncology background, it seemed like a very odd technique for working with distress at the time. I was cynical. However, I had great respect for and trust in my therapy colleague not to try and introduce me to some flaky practice.

I was soon convinced of the benefits of EFT and found it really helpful for working with my personal anxiety, unwanted reactions, stress and distress. I also quickly saw its potential for palliative care patients who, by the very nature of being forced to face their mortality, are dealing with multiple losses, fears, anger, frustrations, indeed the full gamut of human emotions.

But how to introduce such a weird looking treatment mode into the conservative working environment I found myself in at the time? The answer was, slowly. Presenting EFT as a relaxation technique, I taught it to a few patients whom I sensed would be open to it. They found it useful. One of the things I needed to work through, however, was my longstanding fear of being criticised, disrespected and humiliated. Would my colleagues laugh at me? They didn't. Well, not to my face.

Quite soon, however, I recognised that, and personally found, the statements and prescriptiveness of EFT were cumbersome. Many of my patients just did not have the energy and focus for what was entailed.

Then I met Steve Wells and Dr David Lake at a workshop in Sydney. Steve is a psychologist and peak performance consultant and David is a retired general practitioner and psychotherapist. This dynamic duo had simplified the technique and developed SET (Simple Energy Technique) as well as PET (Provocative Energy Technique). They had found that the words and algorithms that I was finding awkward with EFT were actually not necessary to get results. As long as one tapped on the points, this could occur in any order. It was so simple. So, I was hooked and have continued to do as many workshops and coaching sessions with Steve and David as possible. More recently Steve has developed Intention Tapping. This is based on the concept that it is the meaning and attachment to the issue or event that causes suffering rather than the issue/event itself. I have found these techniques invaluable help in my personal self-care/awareness work.

Introducing tapping to patients and their families has been very helpful. It can be used as a tool to help manage distress especially when anxiety and fear are issues. James was such a person for whom tapping was really effective in easing suffering.

I usually introduce tapping as a relaxation technique. Patients often find it empowering as a self-help tool.

Healthcare professionals rightly are keen for a good evidence base for treatments and techniques that they use and recommend. It is thus gratifying to see the expanding evidence base showing tapping does work and with sustained results. It is just not known how.

These are some of the methods, over the years, I have found most useful in pursuing self-awareness. I have used others and there are clearly many, many other techniques and practices that practitioners have found valuable. The key is to explore different modalities and practices to find those that suit you.

Whichever modalities are used, I believe it is vital to commit to on-going self-care and self-awareness. It is our clinical responsibility in helping people achieve the end of life with as much peace, meaning and hope as possible.

Chapter 13

HOPE

Victor Frankl was a psychiatrist who endured the horrors of being a prisoner in a Nazi concentration camp during the Second World War. He chronicled the importance of maintaining hope in dire circumstances in his classic book *Man's Search for Meaning*. As he has said, 'When we are no longer able to change a situation, we are challenged to change ourselves.'

Palliative care aims to foster hope and meaning at the end of life.

There are many books and articles written on the topic of "hope" with attempted definitions. It is not my purpose to try and contribute to that literature. Rather, I want to relate how I have come to see hope towards the end of life. Further, I want to suggest how we might facilitate the blossoming of hope in the presence of suffering and dying. This, I believe, requires our purposeful and conscious presence. Self-awareness makes this possible.

The word "hope" in the context of advanced terminal disease is often taken to mean, the "probability" or "possibility" of cure. Clinicians may collude with this. More and more tests and treatment can reflect the clinician's discomfort in telling the truth and conveying bad news. One may hear the excuse, 'I don't want to take away hope.' But is this really about hope or merely encouraging decisions based on dishonest information? It may reflect the clinician's own fears and reluctance to examine them. Renata's story is an example.

Kaye Herth, a Canadian research nurse, has extensively researched "hope" as an important human response. She has described it as an "Inner power directed toward the enrichment of 'being'". In her many publications, she has identified strategies that foster hope and circumstances that hinder.

Similarly, Snyder, a psychologist, identified three components of hope as: firstly, having goal-orientated thoughts; secondly, strategies are needed to achieve goals; and thirdly, motivation to expend effort to achieve those goals.

As part of her work, Kaye Herth has developed an instrument to measure hope and has written extensively on this. However, hope, like many human attributes, defies definition and is, I contend, impossible to measure.

In the context of working with this indefinable, I find the words of Lois Ramondetta, a gynaecological cancer specialist helpful: '... hope involves a dynamic response to the rough waves on the sea of life' and is 'an active internal process requiring motivational energy.' She goes on to tell us that 'ability to foster hope is ... deeply affected by the external state of affairs and by other individuals.'

Rebecca Solnit wrote in an article in *The Guardian* "On Living in Hard Times", that 'Hope is an embrace of the unknown.' This description also resonates with me.

Over time I have come to believe that hope simply represents emotional and spiritual wellbeing.

With this in mind, it is helpful to identify particular attributes and strategies that do foster hope for each person. Facilitating and encouraging these can allow hope to blossom. I believe that this helps to give life meaning even as death approaches. I hope that the stories I have related demonstrate this.

The following are some of those attributes and strategies.

The presence of meaningful relationships

Feeling connected is a fundamental need for humans. As one approaches the end of life, meaningful relationships can become even more important.

Family and Friends

The importance of relationships with others, friends and/or family are for most people vitally important and give a sense of meaning and hope.

For Alan, for example, his parents' and sisters' support was vital. And he loved being able to spend time with his friends. He was jealous of the things they could do that he couldn't and often rankled at the unfairness. But he told me how important it was for them to come and spend time with him. He knew then they hadn't forgotten him.

Likewise, for Leonie the relationship that she had with her sisters and her children gave her the knowledge that she wouldn't be forgotten. She described a sense of confidence that, although life would be difficult initially for her children, they would be alright.

Animals

Pets play an important part in many peoples' lives. In fact, for some people it is the relationship with an animal that is more important than that with any human.

Maryanne's relationship with Sally was, towards the end of both their lives, paramount. It was the knowledge that Sally was cared for and that she would not be left alone that gave Maryanne the hope for a peaceful death herself.

Places

Our relationship with places that hold special memories can also foster a sense of meaning and hope.

Maryanne needed to visit places in her caravan that had been important to her in her youth.

Alan had a very special relationship with the farm on which he was brought up. It was his last request and hope that he could go there to die.

Light-heartedness and Humour

There is a lot of literature on the value of humour and laughter on mental wellbeing. It has certainly been my experience that with the direst of prognoses towards the end of life, appropriate light-heartedness has an important role.

Maryanne was a woman who often had a twinkle in her eye and would joke with us. She had spent her last months travelling around visiting places from her earlier life. Revisiting them completed her "bucket list" in her words. One morning while she was in the inpatient unit, she asked me how old I was. I was a year or two older than her. With a grin on her face, she looked up at me and said, 'Well, I've completed my "bucket list", how are you going with yours?'

Nancy, likewise, liked to often tease us. Sometimes her sense of humour was a bit alarming when she told us she had needed to use the oxygen while she was having a "fag"! As our mouths fell open, she retorted, 'Only joking!' Another day when we arrived she had put on her rally driving jacket and asked if we wanted to go for a drive. I have a great photo of her posing with a cheeky grin on her face.

Wendy was a woman with very advanced lung disease who came into the inpatient unit for us to try and improve her shortness of breath. She was very sad and miserable on admission. Fortunately, we were able to make her more comfortable with her breathing. She greeted us one morning with what looked like a large glove on her hand. As we started to speak to her out popped a small black teddy bear from the "glove" that "answered" our greeting. Wendy had a huge smile on her face.

Often hospices and palliative care facilities are perceived to be very sad places. Sad things are happening, there can be no doubt. But people are often surprised by the presence of light-heartedness, humour and laughter.

Clear Aims or Goals

When disease cure is no longer possible, there are still things that can be achieved. Clear aims and goals can help achieve a sense of purpose, which in turn increases meaning and hope.

Shirley, who knew she was dying, was clear that she wanted, indeed needed, to hold on until there was a plan for her partner Russell's needs. Being able to achieve that goal gave Shirley a sense of hopefulness and meaning.

Miriam was adamant that she would be cured. However, in her own time, with support and without pressure to change her view, Miriam moved her goal. She was able to see being present at her son's birthday party as a miracle. Only then she was able to express her dreams and hopes for his future.

Daniel was miserable and in pain when he came into the inpatient unit. His pain had been uncontrolled for some weeks. He was desperate, scared and suffering. 'What's going to happen to me? Is this all there is? Am I going to die like this?' he said. He looked at me pleadingly. He was 40 years old and a university lecturer. 'Let's get your pain under control and then we can go from there,' I said. He looked cynical.

By the next day his pain was pretty well controlled. I went in and his whole demeanour had changed. He was comfortable and relaxed. 'I didn't think I was going to be comfortable again,' he said. 'Now I can think about what I can achieve in my last weeks.'

Courage, Determination and Serenity

Personal attributes such as courage, determination and serenity appear to make people more hopeful, certain even, that their goals can be achieved. As those supporting people at the end of life, we need to support and encourage the expression of these qualities. However, this encouragement needs to be balanced with clear and truthful information on which the person can base their goals. A real balancing act at times.

Joe, for instance, was absolutely determined to visit the country of his birth to see his mother before he died. This seemed an impossibility to the healthcare professionals advising him and he knew this. But he was absolutely determined and had the courage to try. When I met him on the flight, I wished I had had an ounce of his serenity. It was a trip that gave great meaning to him as a native of Vietnam and as a son.

And Nancy, the same qualities allowed her to achieve the cruise of her dreams which completed her bucket list, giving her great joy and wonderful memories for both her and her husband, John.

Ability to Recall Positive Moments

These days we are constantly taking photographs. Photographs record our memories so we can look back on them with pleasure. The ability to recall positive moments can give us a sense of the times that were worthwhile, meaningful. Those moments remind us that life itself has meaning. Although photographs can help remind of those times, so too does the sharing of life's stories.

Palliative care services, for this reason, will often help to facilitate this by providing life review or life history services. The facilitator will sit with the person whose life is to be reviewed. They gradually record the events in the way the person wishes them told. This then is transcribed and gives a tangible record and meaningful memento for family after the death of a loved one.

The importance of being able to recall positive memories in the presence of great suffering was never clearer to me than the look of hope in the eyes of Lena.

Lena is part of the family that lost fourteen family members in the devastating tsunami in Samoa in 2009. I worked with a group in Samoa providing emotional support following the tsunami. That was how I first met Lena. She had lost all three of her young children that terrible day. She had been holding her youngest close to her when a shard of glass penetrated him. Such suffering; the loss of her own three dear children and eleven other members of her extended family; this amongst the total devastation that the tsunami wreaked on the beautiful beach village where they lived. How does one survive such loss and grief? There are incredible stories of courage, determination and resilience that followed and Lena's is one of those. A moment that is etched in my heart came some eighteen months later. Lena had become pregnant again and we were visiting her after the birth of her new son. She looked radiant as she showed him to us. She looked into his eyes and then up at us. 'When I look into his eyes,' she said, 'I see my other three children and remember all the wonderful times we had.'

Being able to recall those positive memories gave Lena meaning and hope for the future of her new son.

Having One's Individuality Accepted and Respected

Experiencing unconditional acceptance and respect enhances our sense of self-esteem and worth. It helps to give a sense that we mean something. And this continues until our last breath.

Mark was a great example of this. Towards the end of his life, perhaps for one of the few times ever, he experienced acceptance and love. This gave him the possibility and hope that he might see his son with whom he had lost contact. That hope appeared to give him great joy. He did make contact with him but sadly died before a meeting could be arranged.

Darlene was different. Her "family" was different. Her foster mother and her carer accepted Darlene for who she was. Her hope was reflected in her smile.

Having Beliefs and Religious Practices Respected

Spiritual beliefs can give great solace and hope towards the end of life. One of the roles of healthcare professionals in this context is to support an individual's beliefs and allow their expression without judgement.

I am reminded of Maria who shyly spoke about her sense of connection with the Native American chief and her relief when she felt able to talk about this openly.

Orlando, dying of rabies, asked me whether what was happening to him was a punishment from God. This was in keeping with his strong religious faith, which I certainly didn't share. Putting my belief system to one side and respecting his was really important for both of us. Then, he could deal with his fears and die with hope of forgiveness and redemption.

Knowing that religious rituals at the time of death will be honoured is vital for some. Assurance that such rituals will occur gives some the hope that their passage to a next life will be smoother. There are some traditional and familiar rituals that are requested but some are unique and need to be accommodated if at all possible.

I recall a woman who had certain clothes brought into the inpatient unit that were much too big for her. However, she said that she needed to die in these if possible or to be dressed in them as soon as she died. When, on two occasions, she thought she was about to die she insisted on being dressed in them. However, death did not immediately come. But she was happy to accept reassurance that she would be dressed in them as soon as her transition occurred.

Dealing with Unfinished Business

It is hard to rest easily when there are unresolved issues in one's life. Much of the work of any palliative care team is around helping patients and families to deal with old conflicts and issues; dealing with unfinished business.

Orlando's story illustrates well the need to do this. He was dying, potentially one of the most horrendous deaths imaginable. Once he was confident that his symptoms could be controlled, his suffering centred around the guilt he felt for the affair he had with a woman before he had met his wife. Telling his wife and dealing with that unfinished business allowed a more peaceful death and hope for forgiveness and redemption.

Being Heard

Being heard is, I believe, one of the most important needs of those approaching death. This is true throughout life, of course. But at the sacred time in life that we call dying, we need to know that someone has heard what has been important in our life.

Cathy needed her story of abuse to be heard. Then she could make some sense of her pain.

Pauline's anguish needed to be heard before she could help make plans for her young family. And Leno … How might it have been different for him if I had just given him more attention and listened to his desperation?

Each and every one of us need our stories to be heard. And the more aware I am of my own emotional and spiritual issues, the more I will be able to hear and focus on those that I seek to serve.

My hope for the dying person is that I can support the hope, meaning and self-transcendence that is right for them.

BIBLIOGRAPHY AND FURTHER READING

Chapter 1

Kübler-Ross, Elisabeth, *Working it Through. An Elisabeth Kubler-Ross workshop on Life Death and Transition.* (Touchstone Books, 1997)

Kübler-Ross, Elisabeth, *On Death and Dying.* (New York: MacMillan, 1969)

Chapter 2

Rothschild, Babette, *The Body Remembers.* (Norton Professional Books, 2000)

van der Kolk, Bessell, *The Body Keeps Score.* (Penguin Publishing Group, 2015)

Riva, Giuseppe, 'The neuroscience of body memory: from the self through the space to the others'. *Cortex*, 104, 2018, pp 241-260.

Chapter 4

Marsden, SC, Cabanban, CR, *Rabies:* 'A Significant Palliative Care Issue'. *Progress in Palliative Care*, 2006;14:62-67

Marsden Sue, 'Other Infectious Diseases: Malaria, Rabies, Tuberculosis' in *Textbook of Palliative Medicine and Supportive Care*. Bruera, E, Higginson, IJ, von Gunten, CF, Morita, T, (eds) 2nd Ed (CRC Press, Aug 2016)

Chapter 7

Furth, Gregg M, *The Secret World of Drawings. A Jungian Approach to Healing Through Art*. (Inner City Books, 2002)

Bach, Susan, *Life Paints its Own Span*. (Daimon Verlag, January 1990)

Chapter 11

Eiseley, Loren, The Unexpected Universe. (Harcourt, Brace and World, 1969)

Chapter 12

Nouwen, Henri JM, *The Wounded Healer*. (Image, 1979)

Jung, Carl G, *Man and his Symbols*. (Dell Publishing, 1968)

Watson, Jacob, *Essence: The Emotional Path to Spirit* (O Books John Hunt Pub, 2015)

Johnson, Robert A, *Owning your Own Shadow. Understanding the Dark Side of the Psyche*. (Harper: San Francisco, 1994)

Johnson, Robert A, *Inner Work: Using Dreams and Active Imagination for Personal Growth*. (Harper: San Francisco, 1989)

Durie, Mason, *Whaiora: Maori Health Development*. (Auckland: OUP 1998)

Wells, Steve, *100% Yes The Energy of Success*. (Waterford, 2016)

Wells, Steve and Lake, David, *Enjoy Emotional Freedom*. (Existe Publishing, 2010)

Chapter 13

Frankl, Viktor E, *Man's Search for Meaning*. (Rider, 2008)

Eger, Edith, *The Choice*. (Ebury Pub Rider, 2018)

Herth, Kaye, 'Fostering Hope in Terminally Ill people'. *Journal of Advanced Nursing* 1990:15:1250-1259

Herth, Kaye, 'Development and refinement of an instrument to measure hope'. *Sch Inq Nurs Pract*. Spring 1991:5 (1): 39-51

Herth, Kaye. 'Engendering Hope in the chronically and terminally ill: Nursing Interventions'. *Journal of Hospice and Palliative Medicine*. Sept 1 1995

Ramondetta, Lois, in *Textbook of Palliative Medicine and Supportive Care*. Bruera, E, Higginson, IJ, von Gunten, CF, Morita T, (eds) 2nd Ed (CRC Press, Aug 2016)

Ramondetta, Lois, 'The Importance of Hope'. *Coping Magazine*. 2012, 20-21

Solnit, Rebecca, 'On Living in dark times'. *The Guardian*, 15 July 2016

Groopman, J, *The Anatomy of Hope*. (New York: Random House, 2004)

Cassell, Eric J, *The Nature of Suffering and the Goals of Suffering*. (OUP, 2004)

Cassell, Eric J, *The Nature of Healing. The Modern Practice of Medicine*. (OUP, 2013)

Snyder, CR, *Psychology of hope: You can get there from here*. (New York: Free Press, 2003)

Acknowledgements

For some years I had wanted to write down stories of people I had worked with. Occasionally, I would take pen to paper, but it wasn't until the COVID pandemic lockdowns that much writing happened. What emerged was a first draft of what eventually became this book. At the start I was not sure of my primary focus for writing. I decided that it might, at least, be some sort of record for my children and grandchildren of my experiences in palliative care. It would perhaps provide some sort of explanation of why I was not always as present for them as they would have chosen. I want to acknowledge their forbearance. I also want to thank my husband, John, for his love and total acceptance of me and my absences. He left a large space in my life when he died.

I was unsure whether that first draft would go any further. So, thank you Steve Wells for encouraging the next step and for your help with my commitment and creating deadlines. And thank you to the 100%Yes and FFFF groups for their patience and support.

My thanks to David Lake, Liese Groot-Alberts, Mandy Parris-Piper and Sue Hughes for constructive feedback of the manuscript and encouragement. Janine McVeigh took on the role of coaching this amateur and providing a crash course in writing. Thank you for your patience.

So many friends, colleagues and family have helped with support and honesty. I am not going to name everyone for fear that I miss someone. But thank you all.

I feel very lucky that Mary Egan Publishers agreed to publish 'Thank you, Elisabeth'. To me it seemed like an insurmountable task of getting the project through the many processes required. They have made it smoother. I am particularly grateful to Sophia Egan-Reid for guiding me and communicating with me throughout.

And, of course, I am ever grateful to Elisabeth Kübler-Ross and her team for introducing me to the concept of honest self-awareness and need to "deal with my own shit first".

Lastly but the most important. I salute the courage and authenticity of the many people who have trusted me to work with them at the end of their lives.